Good Fats, Bad Fats

ROSEMARY STANTON

Good Fats,

An Indispensable
GUIDE TO ALL THE FATS
YOU'RE LIKELY TO ENCOUNTER

Bad Fats

MARLOWE & COMPANY
NEW YORK

GOOD FATS, BAD FATS:
An Essential Guide to All the Fats You're Likely to Encounter
Copyright © 1997, 2002 by Rosemary Stanton

Published by
Marlowe & Company
An Imprint of Avalon Publishing Group Incorporated
161 William Street, 16th Floor
New York, NY 10038

Originally published in Australia by Allen & Unwin.
This edition published by arrangement. The publisher would like to thank
Lee Francis for her editorial contributions
to the American edition.

Library of Congress Cataloging-in-Publication Data
Stanton, Rosemary.
Good fats, bad fats : an indispensable guide to all the fats
you're likely to encounter / Rosemary Stanton.
p. cm.
Originally published: St. Leonards, N.S.W. : Allen & Unwin, 1997.
ISBN 1-56924-539-8
1. Lipids in human nutrition—Popular works. 2. Fatty acids
in human nutrition—Popular works. I. Title.

QP751 .S77 2002
612.3'97—dc21   2001055811

9 8 7 6 5 4 3 2 1

Designed by Pauline Neuwirth, Neuwirth & Associates, Inc.

Printed in the United States of America
Distributed by Publishers Group West

❯ For all those who think fat is a foe

CONTENTS

PART III
Food and Your Health

PART IV
Fat-Free Fats

PART V
Dietary Fat and Body Fat

Good Fats, Bad Fats

INTRODUCTION

It's a "fat" race out there and we're sprinting in the wrong direction! Americans are recoiling from fat as if it were poison. Some of us are even suffering from total fat phobia, hating every hint of softness on our bodies and shunning fats at every turn. Fears of cancer, heart disease, stroke, or diabetes have us condemning foods before we've granted them a fair trial. It may surprise you to know, however, that once all the evidence is weighed, not all fats are created equal and not all fats are undesirable.

What do you think of when you hear the word "fat?" Does it conjure up images of rolls of flesh? Perhaps you think of fat in terms of greasy burgers, fried chicken, or gooey chocolate cake. It would be good if we had separate words for different kinds of fat, but we use the term for fats in food as well as for the fats that pad the body. They are intimately related because eating too many fatty foods leads to an increase in body fat. However, just as we all need some body fat, so do we all need some food fats.

Many of us avoid fats because we fear being stricken with ominous diseases they are heavily associated with. On the other end of the spectrum are those of us who gobble vast quantities of the stuff, not giving fat a second thought.

An alarming 61 percent of men and 51 percent of women aged 20 to 74 are overweight or obese.

Consuming vast quantities of fatty foods has become a favorite pastime in America. Many of us eat fat unwittingly because we have little idea which foods contain fat. Fortunately our food industry requires food labels to indicate fat content. However, sometimes labels can confuse or mislead. For instance, a food label may proclaim that its product contains "no cholesterol," but it still may be stuffed with fat.

Many modern foods have more fat than their old-fashioned counterparts. Even a simple hamburger is deceiving. The kind of hamburgers once available, which often seemed quite greasy, averaged about 18 grams of fat. A modern burger, which does not seem to ooze much fat, has at least one and a half times as much fat, sometimes even more.

> **Large quantities of fats are also hidden in unexpected places. For example, who would guess that 1 croissant can have as much fat as nineteen slices of bread, that some muffins have twice the amount of fat as a slice of apple pie, or that a serving of potato chips labeled "light" would have more fat than their traditional counterparts.**

Our grocery store shelves provide us with an enormous range of foods that are high in fat, and most of this fat is a type that nutritionists regard as undesirable. Even foods such as poly- or monounsaturated margarine, which sound as though they have "good" fats, also contain a lot of saturated, or "bad" fats. The food industry tries to make amends—or perhaps just greater profit—by producing an ever-expanding range of foods with reduced fat levels. These are among the fastest-growing lines. Many have less fat than the parent foods that spawned them, but they may still contain unhealthy levels. There is also a rapidly swelling range of fake fats. Some are already being used; others are still on the drawing board. Huge energy resources are being poured into producing fake food ingredients that will supply no energy. In a world where millions of people are starving, it seems almost obscene for our country to use energy resources and technology in this way. While Americans have easy access to a glorious array of foods, others continue to starve for lack of sustenance.

Discussing the issue of fats in food is not simple. Some fats are quite praiseworthy. These essential nutrients have a long and distinguished role in our diet and we avoid them at our peril. The point is not to damn all fats. *Good Fats, Bad Fats* will sort out the truths and the tales in simple, logical terms so you can understand which fats are beneficial and which have no redeeming qualities. This book will go beyond deepening your understanding of fats. It will provide you with the tools you'll need to enhance the strength and vitality your body already possesses.

PART I

The Role of Fats

Before the 20th century, most people thought body fat was good because it represented survival. They also thought highly of foods that contained fat, realizing that those who could afford to eat more of these foods had higher stores of body fat, which was then available to supply energy for the body. In times when foods were scarce, or during illness, a store of fat could mean the difference between survival and death. How times have changed!

REVOLVING VIEWS

The idea that fat is good persists in many areas of the world, especially where an ample food supply is not always assured. In these parts, people still encourage young children to eat more, believing that a plump child is a sign of health and good parenting.

> In some societies, men believe that higher levels of body fat—or, better still, a plump wife—demonstrate their wealth and worth as providers.

Some men in developed countries also believe that the sheer physical space a large, overweight body occupies is an imposing display of power. By contrast, many women feel so insecure about their role that they want to be as thin as possible. In extreme cases, these women develop eating disorders that are partly related to their intense fear of being fat.

Fat and Fertility

In most parts of the world, there is a widespread belief that well-rounded women are more attractive, possibly because they are generally more fertile, and fertility is still prized. The fecundity of well-rounded breasts and hips, and ample thighs, is a major reason many great painters of the past have preferred to portray plumper women. Renoir, Reubens, and Michelangelo would probably have pitied the supermodels of today for their lankiness and lack of flesh.

> **Up to a point, women with more body fat *are* more fertile, although this does not hold for the very obese, who often suffer from infertility.**

Most women who are naturally lean are not infertile, but many of those who reduce their normal body size to become as thin as current fashion demands will stop producing the female hormone estrogen. This is nature's way of preventing pregnancy in a body that does not have enough fat stores to support a healthy pregnancy and period of lactation.

Endocrinologists tell us that girls begin to menstruate when their body fat reaches a level great enough to stimulate an increase in estrogen production. As evidence for this, most plump girls menstruate early, whereas girls who are thinner may not begin menstruation until they are older. Those who are very thin may not menstruate at all.

Others believe menstruation begins when a girl's weight reaches a certain percentage of its genetically destined level, but this theory also depends partly on levels of body fat. All agree that linear growth slows once menstruation begins, when fat deposits develop on breasts, hips, and thighs and the girl matures into womanhood.

Dangerous Obsessions

In a society obsessed with thinness and in which models are praised for their prepubescent low levels of body fat, some girls with normal fat deposits see themselves as having unsightly, abnormal fat bulges. Many think there is something wrong with their bodies and develop a dissatisfaction that can dominate their lives, leading to poor eating habits and low self-esteem. Most reject dietary fat when it comes from sources such as meat and dairy products, although they may continue to nibble on much fattier foods, such as chips and chocolate.

The definition of anorexia nervosa includes the cessation of menstrual periods. Even when the psychological problems that are part of anorexia nervosa have improved, a girl is considered out of danger only when her body fat and estrogen levels are high enough for her menstrual periods to return. From a physiological viewpoint, women need obvious deposits of body fat.

2

NECESSARY FATS

We spend a lot of time trying to banish fats from our bodies. The reality is that without a certain amount of fat, our bodies won't function the way they should. Did you know that fat:

- regulates your body temperature and protects you from extreme heat and cold?
- cushions your internal organs and pads your bones?
- provides a storehouse of energy, especially useful during times of illness or hunger?
- builds and supports your nerve and brain cells?
- aids in absorption of some nutrients?
- influences your production of hormones?

Some fat from the food you eat can be converted into body fat. It's only when you eat too much or too little of it that the body becomes loaded down with excess weight. In addition, the types of fats you indulge in can influence the composition of cell membranes and fat cells. For example, eating a lot of saturated fat gives harder cell membranes and more solid body fat than occurs when the dietary fat is more unsaturated (see Chapter 7).

Bedrocks of Life

The structural components of the human body include bone, muscle, and fat. Fat makes up from 12 to 20 percent of the body weight of a normally sized man, and about 20 to 30 percent of the weight of a normal woman. These are typical levels, and some people are naturally leaner, while others may have higher levels of body fat.

Fat is present as essential fats in your bone marrow and in organs such as your brain, heart, spleen, kidneys, lungs, pancreas, and kidneys. Your body's nervous system is also rich in essential fats. Women have more essential body fat than men because of their fat deposits on breasts, hips, and thighs. These are considered as essential for women because of their role in fertility.

Both men and women also have extra deposits of storage fat in adipose tissue. Some of this tissue is important to protect organs such as your kidneys, and to provide some degree of cushioning over your body. Most is stored beneath the skin as subcutaneous fat.

About 12 percent of men's body weight and 15 percent of women's weight is storage fat.

This fat also provides insulation against the cold, and if you have less of it, you may often feel the cold more intensely, although other factors, such as metabolic rate, are also important to protect the body against cold weather.

We need to stop thinking of all body fat as undesirable. Some is essential. Body fat is a problem only when levels are excessive and especially when the fat is distributed as visceral fat around the abdomen. This can occur in all of us when we eat more than our body can burn for activity. Body fat is essential for normal bone density, especially in women. The risks associated with too little body fat and the problems of an excess of abdominal fat, and the food fats that contribute to it, are discussed later in Part 3.

3

FAT IN FOOD

From a historical perspective, problems due to excess body fat are recent but parallel the increase in foods rich in fat and the decrease in the amount of physical activity. If we go back to earlier times, or to the few remaining areas where people still live in more original conditions, we can easily see why foods that contain fat are highly prized. They are rare. Wild animals have little body fat and virtually the only rich sources of fat are some animal organs such as the liver or brain, as well as the eggs of birds or turtles, nuts, seeds, and grubs. Animal flesh, most fish and other foods from the sea or rivers, native grasses, roots, tubers, and wild fruits and vegetables have little fat. Whales, seals, and other creatures in polar regions are exceptions, but their fat is a beneficial kind that is rich in omega 3 fatty acids (see Chapter 6 for more information on fatty acids).

The Caveman Diet

Humans have inhabited the earth for over 2 million years. Our early ancestors ate a diet that included vegetables, fruit, nuts, seeds, and wild animals. Even in areas where animal flesh may have made up a significant proportion of the diet, the diet was usually low in fat, because wild game meats are lean—typically with about 4 percent fat. Cuts of beef and pork in our supermarkets can have up to 35 percent fat.

MEAT	CALORIES	FAT GRAMS
Antelope, roasted, 3 oz.	128	2
Bear, simmered, 3 oz.	220	11
Beaver, roasted, 3 oz.	180	6
Bison, roasted, 3 oz.	122	2
Boar, wild, roasted, 3 oz.	136	4
Caribou, roasted, 3 oz.	142	4
Deer, roasted, 3 oz.	134	3
Moose, roasted, 3 oz.	114	1
Rabbit, wild, stewed, 3 oz.	147	3
Squirrel, roasted, 3 oz.	147	4

In primitive societies, fat in large quantities is hard to find. For this reason, when an animal was killed, the brain and liver were so highly regarded that they were reserved for the most important members of the tribe. These foods caused no problems because the total diet was so low in fat. The relatively high fat content of some fish, reptiles, moths, and grubs did not contribute much total fat overall because those foods were not eaten excessively. The exception occurred in the Arctic Circle, where whales and seal blubber were consumed in large quantities.

Essential fatty acids, which your body must get from food, are found in the fats of nuts, seeds, eggs, and in most river, lake, and saltwater fish. Grasses, wild vegetables, and the lean flesh of animals, birds, and reptiles also boost the intake of essential fatty acids, even though these foods contain only relatively small quantities of fat. Foods such as chocolate, potato chips, and fried foods, on the other hand, have a lot of fat but little or no essential fatty acids.

Cultural Evolutions

In general, before animals were domesticated and packaged processed foods were readily available, only about 10 percent of the day's energy came from fat. In most affluent countries, fat intake is now about four times this level, supplying 30 to 40 percent of energy. Average total energy intake in affluent countries has not increased to any extent, but its composition has changed dramatically from being high in carbohydrates to being high in fat.

For some cultures, a diet rich in fat serves an important physiological purpose. The Inuit people (Eskimos), who once consumed large quantities of fatty cold-water fish, whales, and seals, have a natural food supply that is rich in fat. Living in extremely cold conditions, this dietary fat was essential to increase body fat levels to provide insulation against the harsh weather conditions. The fats from these cold-water sea creatures are also rich in particular types of omega 3 polyunsaturated fatty acids, which may protect against heart disease and some cancers.

In stark contrast to the food supply available throughout millions of years of history over most parts of the earth, the modern Western food supply is saturated with vast quantities of fat.

You can't see much of the fat we eat, as it comes from fats and oils already present in processed foods.

Today, fats and oils used in prepared food and home cooking make up about half of our fat intake, followed by meat and dairy products as the next major sources.

In parts of Asia and the Middle East, fat consumption is also increasing rapidly, in line with affluence. Health authorities preach the virtues of eating more fresh foods, with less fat, but in every society, as people become more affluent, they discard their healthy low-fat food habits for processed convenience foods. For example, in Japan, fat intake has accelerated over the last twenty years, rising from 10 percent of energy to 25 percent. Over the same period, subcutaneous body fat has more than doubled.

Singaporeans show similar trends, and 25 percent of the population now has excessively high levels of body fat, where once it was rare to find anyone in this category. Even in our country, where there is a lot of adverse publicity about dietary fat and a plethora of fat-reduced foods, the fat intake continues to climb.

> **The excessive amount of saturated fat we eat contributes to the $105 billion the U.S. pays out for costs associated with heart disease.**

Our consumption of low-fat products has also increased, but it doesn't make up for the massive influx of fat from fast foods.

Life in the Fast Food Lane

While women today have more career options than at any other time in history, many of them find themselves still responsible for most food decisions, from shopping to cooking to cleaning up afterward. Advertisers realize how processed and ready-prepared foods appeal to women who juggle a career, housework, and children. It's understandable why people across the world have embraced the concept of drive-thru windows and hand-delivered meals. The name says it all: "fast food." Sales figures clearly indicate that our consumption of fast foods, and therefore our fat intake, is steadily rising.

> **Forty-six percent of our food dollar is spent on meals and snacks prepared outside of the home, with fast foods making up approximately one-third of this amount.**

Most people eat fast foods because they are cheap, convenient, and save busy people the trouble of having to think about what to eat. The TV commercials are wholesome and lively and the premises are clean and convenient. Perhaps more important, the bright decor and "free" toys with every meal are designed to keep our children content.

Few people eat these foods for the taste experience. For many of us, our favorite food memories go back to our mother's home cooking, usually associated with good quality fresh ingredients mixed with a long session in the kitchen and a lot of love.

Old-style home-cooked foods, however, are not fat free. Fat carries and develops flavor, and all good cooks are aware of this. Frying is especially good at causing chemical changes that add to flavor. For example, you cannot get as much flavor by steaming an onion as you can when the onion is fried. But at least, when you cook your foods from scratch, you are aware of the quantity of fat you are adding.

> It's difficult to be aware of the high fat content of foods someone else has prepared. The fact that fast foods are convenient and high in fat is an unfortunate coincidence. The misfortune lies in what those types of fat can do to our bodies.

4

LIVE LONG AND PROSPER

In the beginning there was breast milk. It is a relatively high-fat food, supplying more than half its calories from fat. Most infants triple their birth weight in the first twelve to fifteen months of life, and such a rapid growth rate needs the concentrated source of calories that fat can provide.

Once growth stops, and certainly by the time we reach adulthood, we need much less dietary fat. The exact percentage of our calories that should come from fat is not certain. Before animals were domesticated to provide milk and meat, and long before processed foods dominated the diet, most human populations got about 10 percent of their energy from fat. That may well be an ideal level.

Our average intake is estimated as 37 percent. Most experts recommend we eat 30 percent or less of our daily calories as fat. No study has ever shown this figure to be optimal; it is set as a goal because it is considered to be potentially achievable within the food environment of developed countries.

Greek Lessons

We can build a good case that there is no *single* desirable level of dietary fat.

> The longest life expectancy occurred in Greece up to the 1960s. The Greek diet up to that time had at least 45 percent of its calories from fat.

By contrast, the longest-living people in the 1990s were the Japanese, and their diet had approximately 25 percent of calories from fat, although most of the elders who contributed to the statistics for long life expectancy would have had even lower levels of fat (approximately 15 percent of energy) for most of their lives. It is also worth noting that up until the 1960s the Greeks lived longer than the Japanese do now. Since the Greeks reduced their total fat intake and substituted more saturated fats and processed foods for their previously olive oil–dominated diet, their incidence of coronary heart disease has increased and their length of life has decreased.

Life Expectancies

Genetics play a heavy hand in your life expectancy, but so does lifestyle. Many dietary habits are greatly influenced by culture. Here are the top 10 countries rated by the World Health Organization for "full health," which includes total lifetime expectancy without disabilities.

Country	Years
Japan	74.5
Australia	73.2
France	73.1
Sweden	73.0
Spain	72.8
Italy	72.7
Greece	72.5
Switzerland	72.5
Monaco	72.4
Andorra	72.3

We rate at number 24 under this system, with an average of 70 years of healthy life.

There seems to be much better evidence that it is not the *quantity* of fat that is important, but the *quality*. We also need to consider other protective factors from foods that may be making the major contribution to low death rates from both heart disease and cancers.

The Greek diet was rich in monounsaturated fat, mainly from olive oil and nuts. Both these foods are also rich in a wide variety of antioxidants that prevent the harmful effects produced when fats oxidize (see Chapter 13 for more details). Fruits, vegetables, legumes, red wine, and tea are also excellent sources of protective substances. Except for red wine, the Japanese diet and most other healthful diets contain plenty of these protective plant-based foods.

By contrast, our Western diet is rich in saturated fats, which we know can lead to fatty deposits in the arteries. Over the past few years, the consumption of polyunsaturated fats has also risen. These fats are essential in small quantities but can oxidize readily in your arteries (and in the frying pan), causing damage.

> **Polyunsaturates can lower the "bad" LDL cholesterol, but more is not better, as large quantities can also reduce levels of the "good" HDL cholesterol in blood.**

Back to Basics

The idea that all body fat and fats in food are inherently bad for you is wrong. For the very young and the very old, nutrient requirements are high.

> **There is also plenty of evidence that fats from foods containing other nutrients necessary for growing children should not be shunned.**

For example, a low-fat diet in childhood is accompanied by low levels of preformed vitamin A. A lack of dietary fat also reduces the absorption of beta-carotene, which the body can convert into vitamin A in older children and adults. This is a major reason that young children should be given regular milk rather than skim milk, which lacks fat. Skim milk is fine for older children and adults, who do not rely on milk as a major source of nutrients.

Elderly people may also need more dietary fat. Nutritional deficiencies and weight loss are especially problematic for the very old, and a good source of calories, such as from fat, may be protective. It may therefore be inappropriate to tell the whole community to eat less fat, when at both extremes of age the calories fat supplies play a vital role. It makes sense for children and elders to consume foods that supply fats along with other nutrients.

This rules out promoting fatty chips, pastries, cakes, and many fast foods and deep-fried products as good foods for kids and seniors. High-fat but nutritious foods such as avocado, nuts or nut butters, seeds, fatty fish, eggs, good quality meats, milk, cheese, and yogurt are more suitable.

PART II

Kitchen Chemistry 101

Put aside everything you know or heard about chemistry for a moment. Sweep away images of test tubes, Petri dishes, and microscope slides. Instead, imagine your kitchen. That's right! Your kitchen is where you witness chemistry in action every day. When you boil water, bake brownies, or freeze last night's lasagna, you are setting into motion a veritable earthquake of molecules.

5

THE FUNCTIONS OF FAT IN YOUR BODY

Your body makes body fat from food fat. As we've mentioned earlier, fatty acids (a form of fat) that your diet supplies you with are essential to your body. Fatty acids, phospholipids, and cholesterol form part of the structure of the membranes around every one of your cells. Phospholipids are also involved in blood clotting, and cholesterol is needed to make bile for digestion of fats. Without cholesterol your body wouldn't be able to manufacture some hormones, including sex hormones. And that's just for starters. Fats and fatty acids:

- provide calories, especially important for babies, the elderly, and in anyone where unwanted weight loss is a concern
- are used in nerve, brain, and skin cells and also in the retina of the eye
- are used to make prostaglandins, hormonelike substances that are involved in controlling inflammation, blood pressure, and other reactions in your body
- assist in the absorption of beta-carotene (one type of carotenoid), which your body converts to vitamin A
- help the body to process other carotenoids, which may be valuable in preventing many cancers
- delay the emptying of your stomach, giving you a feeling of fullness after eating. While this can be an undesirable feature of an exceptionally fatty meal, it helps regulate the release of food from your stomach

into the small intestine over several hours after a
meal, preventing the rapid return of hunger

▸ are needed to make body fat for cushioning and insu-
lating your organs

6

THE FUNCTIONS OF FAT
IN YOUR FOOD

Fats in foods are referred to as "lipids" and they are made up of a mixture of different substances, including:

- triglycerides
- phospholipids
- sterols, such as cholesterol
- lipoproteins (combinations of fat and protein)

In the following chapters we will help you understand these fats more fully by providing you with a glimpse into the amazing framework each one is built upon.

Triglycerides and Fatty Acids

Triglycerides are the most prevalent fats, making up more than 95 percent of your body fat. They consist of a glycerol molecule, which is chemically identified as an alcohol. In addition to the glycerol molecule, triglycerides contain 3 fatty acids. Most triglycerides contain more than one type of fatty acid, usually saturated or unsaturated, which we'll discuss in Chapters 7, 8, and 9.

> When glycerol is without its fatty acid partners, it's sometimes used in icing and sweets to stop sugar molecules crystallizing. It is also used in lipstick. Various types of glycerides are used in place of fats in fat-reduced products.

The Raising of a Fatty Acid

Fatty acids contain a chain of carbon atoms—sometimes as many as 35, although most common fatty acids have between 4 and 22 carbon atoms.

When the ends of the fatty acids join a triglyceride, they are properly referred to as "fats."

The Pattern Is the Key

Fatty acids are arranged in a variety of different ways within triglycerides. Food processing can cause them to reassemble. For example, fatty acids in oil may change position if the oil is processed into mayonnaise or margarine. The arrangement of the fatty acids influences physical characteristics such as the melting point of the processed product.

> Some medical researchers have also found that changes in the arrangement of the fatty acids may alter the way the fat is used in the body. If future research confirms that this is important, dietary guidelines may recommend unprocessed fats in foods like olive oil or nuts in preference to processed fats like those in spreads.

Oils

Triglycerides that contain at least two saturated fatty acids are usually solid at room temperature, whereas those with two unsaturated fatty acids are oils at room temperature. When nutritionists refer to the fat content of the diet, however, they include all types of fats and oils.

Cold-pressed oils, made by squashing the oil-rich fruit of olives, the seeds of grapes or sunflowers, or legumes such as peanuts or soybeans, probably retain their original and most desirable arrangement of fatty acids, along with their rich supply of different antioxidants. Oils that are extracted with a chemical solvent and processed into spreads, shortenings, or fats used for frying may become rearranged and lose some of their original antioxidants. Currently it's unclear how much the way fats are produced influences our health. Some argue that once fats are consumed, the first stage in digestion is to split the fatty acids away from the glycerol part of the molecule, making their original arrangement less important.

Oils extracted using a chemical solvent usually have an antioxidant added to stop them from going rancid. The *quantity* of antioxidant in cold-pressed or solvent-extracted oils is similar, but the cold-pressed products may have many antioxidants rather than a single variety of added antioxidant. Again, no one can say for certain whether this matters, but many researchers believe the real value of olive oil lies with its diversity of antioxidants as much as with the type of fatty acids it contains.

As mentioned earlier, there are various types of fatty acids. To simplify the task of classifying them, fatty acids are usually divided into the following classes:

- saturated
- monounsaturated
- polyunsaturated

They are discussed in detail in the chapters that follow.

7

SATURATED FATS

As you'll recall, fatty acids are basically a string of carbon atoms. Those carbon atoms are usually partnered with hydrogen atoms. It's the number of carbon atoms and how hydrogen atoms cling to them that distinguishes one fatty acid from another.

> **Saturated fatty acids have as many hydrogen atoms as possible. In fact, they are said to be "saturated" with hydrogen.**

There are many different saturated fatty acids. They are identified chemically by the number of carbon atoms they contain. For example, palmitic acid, one of the most common saturated fats, is chemically known as C16:0, meaning that it has 16 carbon atoms in its chain and no double bonds. Stearic acid, another common saturated fatty acid, has 18 carbon atoms and its chemical ID is C18:0.

Playing the Numbers

Nutritionists know that every gram of fat contributes 9 calories per gram, a level more than twice that for carbohydrates and protein, which each supply 4 calories per gram. Some researchers believe that saturated fats may contain more than 9 calories per gram. At this stage, however, 9 calories is the accepted figure for all fats. As described in Chapter 10, some fatty acids should have a greater role in your daily diet than others, but all fats are high in calories. This is one reason a diet high in fat easily leads to excess body weight.

A Fat Veggie?

You might assume that saturated fats come only from animal sources. In fact, saturated fats are found in both animal and plant foods. Vegetable foods such as coconut, palm, and palm kernel oils, and cocoa butter (used for making chocolate), are rich in saturated fats.

> On the average, Americans ate 4.2 lbs. of butter and 8.3 lbs. of margarine. (1998 data)

When vegetable fats and oils are processed into solid or semi-solid fats for spreads or as shortenings for making pastries and cakes, some of those that were once largely unsaturated acquire extra hydrogen atoms to become saturated fats. This process is called hydrogenation. It increases the stability of the fat so that it does not go rancid so easily, but it also changes the nature of the fat to one that is potentially harmful. When a food label lists "hydrogenated vegetable oil" among the ingredients, the product will have a higher content of saturated fat than the original oil from which it was made.

> Many commercially fried foods claiming to have been cooked in vegetable oil have usually been cooked in a vegetable oil that was first hydrogenated into a saturated fat. Some of these fats are much higher in saturated fat than beef dripping or lard, but consumers mistakenly believe they are better because the label describes them as "vegetable."

There are also other fatty acids with odd numbers of carbon atoms, but these occur less often in foods.

Saturated fatty acids	Major Food Sources
Acetic acid	vinegar (provides its sharp taste and odor)
Propionic acid	added to bakery and dairy products to inhibit mold
Butyric acid	butterfat (small amount)
Caproic acid	butterfat (small amount)
Caprylic acid	coconut oil
Capric acid	palm oil and goat's milk
Lauric acid	coconut oil (notorious for raising cholesterol)
Myristic acid	coconut oil (notorious for raising cholesterol)
Palmitic acid	palm oil, beef, butter, lard, chocolate, margarines (notorious for raising cholesterol)
Stearic acid	red meats, butter, lard, chocolate
Arachnic acid	peanut oil (small amount)
Behenic acid	peanuts (small amount)
Lignoceric acid	peanut oil (small amount)

As you can see, acetic acid is the main component of vinegar, not a product you would normally consider as "fatty." Acetic, propionic, butyric, caproic, and caprylic acids are all soluble in water and none of them are "fatty" in the usual sense of the word. In the technical language of chemists, however, they are fatty acids.

Acetic, propionic, and butyric acids are usually found in your colon. They are made by bacteria that ferment dietary fiber, and butyric acid serves as a fuel for cells in the bowel. There is a growing body of evidence that butyric acid (also called butyrate) protects against bowel cancer.

Chain Links

The length of the carbon-atom chain determines the characteristics and absorbability of fats. The lengths of chains commonly fall under three classifications.

Short-Chain Fatty Acids

Each of the fatty acids with up to eight carbon atoms in its chain is called a *short-chain* fatty acid, although some people feel that caprylic acid fits better as a medium-chain fatty acid. They are found only in small quantities in most foods. Dairy products are the major source, and butter has a high content of butyric acid, as its name suggests.

Medium-Chain Fatty Acids

Fatty acids with between eight and fourteen carbon atoms are generally called *medium-chain* fatty acids. Caprylic (depending on your classification), capric, lauric acid, and myristic acid are found in a range of foods. Goat's milk has a high content of capric acid, with four to seven times as much of this fatty acid as human milk and about three times the level found in cow's milk. Lauric acid is the major fatty acid in coconut. Myristic is coconut's second most common fatty acid and is also present in fairly high quantities in dairy products like cow's and goat's milk. Some people classify myristic acid as a long-chain acid.

Oils containing medium-chain triglycerides (MCT) are made from coconut oil and consist mainly of caprylic and capric saturated fatty acids. Your body breaks them down more easily than it does other triglycerides. Once they are absorbed, the portal vein blood carries them straight to your liver, where they can provide you with a quick source of energy, if needed.

Not very long ago, researchers assumed that medium-chain triglycerides had little effect on blood cholesterol, but we know better today. Two of the most notable acids to be implicated in raising blood cholesterol are lauric and myristic acids.

Some athletes mistakenly assume that MCTs have advantages over other fats in providing a ready source of energy to enhance their performance. There is little evidence to support this and nothing to justify the high prices sometimes charged for these fats. One study showed that MCT oils can easily end up as abdominal fat. Most athletes need more carbohydrates to supply energy, not fat.

Long-Chain Fatty Acids

All the fatty acids with more than 14 carbon atoms are called *long-chain* fatty acids and they are the predominant type of saturated fat in most foods. High sources include almost all fast foods; most commercial fried foods; red meats; chicken; dairy products such as butter, cream, cheese, yogurt, whole milk, and margarine; processed foods such as pastries, cakes, cookies, crackers; and chocolate.

Saturated fatty acids contribute energy and are important for growth in young animals and human babies. Too many saturated fats are undesirable, however, as they lead to an increase in blood cholesterol and blood clotting and are strongly correlated with coronary heart disease and type 2 diabetes.

Chocolate

Chocolate and beef fat are both high in the saturated fatty acid stearic acid. This does not increase blood levels of LDL cholesterol, a point often made by confectionery manufacturers. There are several other facts that are important, however. Chocolate is also rich in palmitic acid which *can* raise LDL cholesterol levels. There is also some evidence that stearic acid increases the tendency of blood to form clots, although not all recent research confirms this. An analysis of chocolate reveals that many chocolates contain little cocoa butter and a lot of palm and palm kernel oil. Sadly for chocolate lovers, there is little that can be said in favor of the fats in chocolate, except that they taste appealing to most people. Chocolate lovers will be delighted in some new studies that show chocolate contains some antioxidants. Whether they are as protective in the body as they seem to be in the test tube is not yet known.

8

Monounsaturated fats

Earlier we mentioned that each carbon atom in saturated fats go hand in hand with hydrogen atoms. In the case of monounsaturated fats, two side-by-side carbon atoms are missing their hydrogen partners. That absence causes those two lonely carbon atoms to strengthen the bond between them. They form what is called a "double bond." When this occurs, a monounsaturated fat is born.

Monounsaturated Fats and Cholesterol

There is some professional debate on the effects of monounsaturated fat on blood cholesterol. They do not increase LDL ("bad") cholesterol levels and make a good substitute for saturated fat or refined carbohydrates, as they do not reduce HDL ("good") cholesterol. So everyone agrees that monounsaturated fatty acids are "good guys" and a far healthier choice than saturated fats.

Monounsatured Fatty Acids	Major Food Sources
Palmitoleic acid	Seafood, turkey, chicken, beef
Oleic acid	Olive, peanut and canola oils, margarine, nuts, fish, eggs, avocado

Monounsatured Fatty Acids	Major Food Sources
Elaidic acid (trans fat)	Margarine, shortening, hydrogenated fats
Erucic acid	Rapeseed oil

The most common monounsaturated fatty acid is oleic acid. Oleic acid is also the most widespread of all fatty acids, and is the most dominant type in all kinds of meat, eggs, dairy products, lard, dripping, and all soft margarines except those labeled "polyunsaturated."

Erucic acid comes from rapeseeds, a vegetable crop that grows easily and crops heavily. However, erucic acid has an unfortunate effect. It enters the cells, including those in the heart muscle, and accumulates there due to its very slow rate of oxidation. Plant geneticists have developed a rapeseed with only 2 percent erucic acid which we commonly know as canola oil. It contains mainly oleic acid but also some alpha-linolenic acid. Theoretically, it looks even better than olive oil, although it does not have the history of use, the flavor, or variety of antioxidants found in olive oil.

White Knights

Monounsaturated fatty acids are generally considered the "good guys" because they do not increase blood cholesterol levels. The exception is elaidic acid, a fatty acid formed when vegetable oils are processed to make spreads. Elaidic acid is called a trans-fatty acid because of the way its molecule lies. It does not occur in nature.

9

POLYUNSATURATED FATS

Polyunsaturated fatty acids (sometimes called PUFA) have more than one double bond between carbon atoms in their chain. They fit into two major classes: omega 6, written as n–6; and omega 3, written as n–3. These basic fatty acids are converted in the body to hormonelike substances called prostaglandins, thromboxanes, and prostacyclins. The relationship between omega 3 and 6 positions is important because the types of prostaglandins made from each have opposite but potentially complementary roles. Too much of one kind in relation to the quantity of the other can alter inflammatory reactions in your body's tissues and interfere with the stickiness of blood cells, changing how much or how little blood cells will form clots.

The Omegas

In the typical American diet, the ratio of omega 6 to omega 3 fatty acids has become unbalanced, largely because we are eating more of an omega 6 polyunsaturated fatty acid called linoleic acid. This fatty acid is essential in small quantities, which is how it would normally be consumed in a diet of natural whole foods.

Omega 3 fatty acids have a more limited distribution in the food chain and the balance between the two types has suffered as a result. Vegetables, some seeds, and canola and soybean oils contain small quantities of an omega 3 fatty acid called alpha-linolenic acid (ALA), while fish and other seafoods and breast milk are excellent sources of very long-chain omega 3s.

Linoleic acid is the major polyunsaturated fatty acid in American diets. Intake has risen steadily as polyunsaturated margarines and oils have become more popular. Major sources include margarines and vegetable oils such as corn, soybean, safflower, sunflower, cottonseed, and sesame. Walnuts, pecans, and Brazil nuts have more polyunsaturated fat than other nuts, which are higher in monounsaturated fatty acids.

Polyunsaturated fatty acids	*Major Food Sources*
Omega 3	
Alpha-linolenic acid	flaxseeds, canola, soybean, walnut and wheat germ oil, nuts, seeds
EPA and DHA	breast milk, fish, shellfish
Omega 6	
Linoleic acid	corn, soybean, safflower, sunflower, and sesame oils
Arachidonic acid	liver, kidney, turkey, fish

10

ESSENTIAL FATTY ACIDS (EFAs)

Your body is a miraculous machine that has the ability to manufacture most of the types of fatty acids that it needs to hum along. However, there are some fatty acids—called essential fatty acids—that your body can't make. Therefore, they must be supplied by food. They are called:

- linoleic acid, which is part of a family of the omega 6 family of fats
- alpha-linolenic acid, or ALA, which is part of the omega 3 family

Your body can use these fatty acids as building blocks for all the other essential fatty acids. Essential fatty acids contribute to the structure of the walls around every cell in your body, and are especially important to cells within your brain and nervous system. These fatty acids also make prostaglandins, hormonelike substances involved in controlling inflammation, blood pressure, and other body reactions. ALA can help the body make other members of the omega 3 family, including eicosapentaenoic acid (EPA) and docosahexaenoic acid (DHA). If you eat fish or other seafood, you get EPA and DHA "ready-made." They are also found in breast milk and are especially important for the eye and the brain. Studies also link them with the prevention of heart disease, some types of arthritis, and certain cancers.

> The content of essential fatty acids in any fat is always
> important, but don't be fooled. You can't tell just by look-
> ing at foods whether they are good sources of fatty acids.

For example, the visible fat on meat and the fats used in
most processed foods are low in essential fatty acids, whereas
other foods that don't appear fatty at all, such as vegetables and
fish, may be important sources of essential fat.

Essential Fatty Acids	*Major Food Sources*
Omega 6	
Linoleic acid	seeds, walnuts, pecans, grains, leafy vegetables, vegetable oils (corn, sesame, sunflower, soybean)
Omega 3	
Alpha-linolenic acid	flaxseeds, nuts, vegetable oils (canola, soybean, wheat germ)
EPA and DHA	breast milk, shellfish, all fish (especially salmon, sardines, herring)

Breast milk is particularly rich in DHA, which supports the
functioning of the retina and the brain. Studies show that
babies who are breastfed have sharper vision for the first eight
or nine months of life, compared with those given formula. For
more information on this vital nutrient see Chapter 18.

> The essential omega 6 and omega 3 fatty acids must be
> in perfect harmony with each other. For example, too
> much of the omega 6s relative to omega 3s will make
> your blood clot too readily, whereas the opposite will
> cause you to bleed excessively after a cut.

This was first noticed in the Inuit people, who have a very high intake of omega 3 fatty acids from fish, seal flesh, and whale blubber. While their arteries were clot free, they bled for a longer time after a cut.

The Gold Standard

Your body isn't able to make omega 3s or omega 6s from its own resources. Your body also cannot change an omega 3 to an omega 6 or vice versa. In fact, they both compete for the same enzymes to complete their families. It's best to try to maintain a healthy balance of these fats through diet.

The "gold standard" food that offers an ideal balance? Breast milk. While it's not a very realistic option for most people, it's vitally important for babies. It's worth noting that it has about five times as many omega 6 fatty acids as omega 3s. A ratio of up to 6:1 is considered acceptable for adults.

> However, you should feel heartened to know that if you eat fish twice a week, you are giving your body a balanced formula of omega 6s and omega 3s.

On the other hand, if you eat a diet that includes a lot of polyunsaturated oils and margarines, which are rich in linoleic acid, you could have 14 to 40 times as much omega 6 as omega 3 fatty acids.

If fish makes a rare appearance on your plate, your body will rely on making the essential EPA and DHA from its parent compound, alpha-linolenic acid (ALA). Linoleic acid and ALA both require the same enzyme to grow. If you overload on linoleic acid, it will use up all the enzyme and ALA won't be able to convert to other essential fatty acids.

> If you, like many Americans, lack omega 3 fatty acids, you may be tempted to include oils such as canola in

your diet. However, your body recognizes it as alpha-
linolenic acid, and it's beneficial only if your diet does not
also contain a lot of polyunsaturated products.

The easiest solution to these problems is to use an omega 9
oil, such as olive, in preference to a polyunsaturated oil, and to
eat plenty of vegetables as well as fish or other seafoods regularly. Olive oil does not enter the competition and so does not
prevent the alpha-linolenic acid in plant foods such as flaxseeds
and canola being converted to the truly essential longer-chain
fatty acids. A deficiency in omega 6 fatty acids is usually a
problem only if you try to avoid all fats.

11

PROSTAGLANDINS AND EICOSANOIDS

Eicosanoids is a general term that embraces substances that have hormonelike actions in the body. They are called:

▶ prostaglandins
▶ thromboxanes
▶ leukotrienes

These substances control blood pressure, blood clotting, the reproductive cycle, and inflammatory reactions and are vital for life and health. They are made from essential fatty acids. The thromboxanes and leukotrienes derived from the omega 3 and omega 6 fatty acids must be in balance or you can have problems with blood clotting and inflammatory reactions. If you suffer with some types of arthritis, an inflammation of the joints, or your blood clots too readily, more of the omega 3 fatty acids and less of the omega 6s can help. In practice, this means eating more fish and vegetables and less margarine and polyunsaturated vegetable oils.

Here are the fatty acids that make up eicosanoids and the foods in which you can find them:

Dihomo-gamma-linolenic acid (DGLA)	evening primrose oil
Arachidonic acid (AHA)	liver, kidney, turkey, fish, meat
Eicosapentaenoic acid (EPA)	fish

Evening Primrose Oil

The major fatty acid in evening primrose oil is gamma-linolenic acid (GLA), a member of the omega 6 family, often promoted as an essential supplement. It has some uses, especially for children who lack an enzyme called delta-6-desaturase. These children may develop a particular type of eczema in early infancy. Until their bodies begin to produce adequate amounts of the enzyme, a regular supplement of evening primrose oil, with its high content of GLA, can help their eczema. Since only a few forms of eczema are related to GLA, only a few can be helped by supplements of evening primrose oil.

> **Evening primrose oil has been touted as being a remedy for menopausal or premenstrual problems although there is no proof that it has any greater effect than a placebo.**

It is hard to understand the rationale for prescribing evening primrose oil to a population that already has high levels of linoleic acid, which is converted to GLA, the major fat in evening primrose oil. The only rationale would be a lack of the delta-6-desaturase enzyme, and there is no evidence of this. In fact, the type of prostaglandins that dominate blood clotting show that you might be better off without so many omega 6 fatty acids.

Research into evening primrose oil and other oils rich in omega 6 fatty acids, such as borage and blackberry, is continuing, and they may turn out to have some unforeseen use. Some keen salespeople often try to sell evening primrose oil as a source of omega 3 fatty acids. You should question their knowledge of the subject of essential fatty acids.

12

PHOSPHOLIPIDS

As we mentioned earlier, triglycerides are the most prevalent fats in your body. Although phospholipids make up less than 5 percent of body fat, they are vital to your cells. They are very similar to triglycerides, but instead of having 3 fatty acids, they have 2. That missing acid is replaced by a complex molecule that contains phosphorus.

Phospholipids are needed for the structure of your nerves and muscles. They are water soluble at one end and fat soluble at the other. This makes them excellent detergents.

Lecithin

The best-known phospholipid is lecithin. It makes up about 30 percent of an egg yolk and it is this property of egg yolk that can stop fat and water from separating. Lecithin is used widely as a food additive to stop oily components from separating out of foods such as Hollandaise sauce, dressings, mayonnaise, desserts, and peanut butter.

> You can find lecithin supplements in most health food stores. However, your body makes its own lecithin to transport fats, so that taking extra quantities has no special benefit.

Claims that taking lecithin will reduce cholesterol are unproven. It also has no effect in reducing body weight. Although it is a fat, few people are likely to take enough of it to increase their weight.

13

STEROLS AND CHOLESTEROL

The most notorious member of the sterol family of fats is a waxy substance called cholesterol. Cholesterol is an essential part of the structure of all cell membranes and is also used for making the bile acids you need to absorb fats as well as vitamin D and some hormones.

Your body does not need a ready-made source of cholesterol since it can be made in your liver and in some of your cells.

> **At this very moment, your body is making cholesterol—it can make up to 1000 mg a day.**

If your diet is high in saturated fat, you may be making more cholesterol than you need. In your body, cholesterol is carried through the blood attached to lipoproteins (combinations of fats and proteins). If a high level of cholesterol is being carried on low-density lipoproteins (LDL), some cholesterol may be deposited in the walls of your arteries. If these deposits are in your coronary arteries and become oxidized, they break off in pieces known as foam cells. These can block the artery so that blood cannot get through, causing a heart attack.

Antioxidants

Some antioxidants may prevent this oxidation reaction occurring. Products such as olive oil, which can have thirty to forty different antioxidants, can help to prevent this reaction. Fruits, vegetables, whole grains, nuts, red wine, and tea are also excellent sources of protective antioxidants. The inclusion of olive oil and most of these foods in the diet may explain why people in Mediterranean countries have such low rates of coronary heart disease even though their average cholesterol levels are similar to those in populations in countries such as ours.

Although about 80 percent of the cholesterol in your body is made in your liver, some is also available, ready-made, from animal foods. A very high intake of these can increase your blood cholesterol levels, but this usually occurs only when the diet is also high in saturated fat. While only foods derived from animals contain cholesterol, not all of them are harmful. For example, shellfish contain cholesterol but studies have shown that eating seafood regularly won't increase bad LDL cholesterol, and some have reported a favorable increase in good HDL cholesterol.

> **Egg yolks can raise cholesterol, but only if the diet is high in saturated fat. The American Heart Association approves the consumption of up to 4 eggs a week. On the average, Americans eat approximately 3 eggs a week.**

If you ate daily helpings of fatty bacon and fried eggs served on buttered toast, your blood-cholesterol levels would almost certainly increase because the ready-made cholesterol was being served with a hearty supply of saturated fat. If your blood cholesterol level is high, you should restrict saturated fats in your diet rather than foods containing cholesterol. A health claim of "cholesterol free" on the label means the product has less than 2 milligrams of cholesterol and less than 2 grams of saturated fat per serving. The chart below shows you how some common foods measure up.

The Cholesterol Content of Foods

Food	Cholesterol content (in milligrams)
Baked Goods	
Cake, angel food, 1 slice, 1 oz.	0
Cake, chocolate, without frosting, 3 oz.	55
Dairy	
Cheese, 1 oz. cheddar	30
Cheese, cottage, 1 cup. 1% fat	10
Cream, sour, 1 tbs.	5
Ice cream, 1 cup	60
Milk, breast, 8 oz.	40
Milk, colostrum, approx. 4 oz.	30
Milk, skim, 1 cup	5
Milk, 1 cup, whole	35
Yogurt, plain, low-fat, 8 oz.	15
Yogurt, whole fat, 8 oz.	30
Eggs	
Egg, whole	210
Egg, white	0
Fats	
Butter, 1 tbs.	30
Mayonnaise, 1 tbs.	10
Meats: Beef, Lamb, Pork, Poultry	
Beef, roasted, lean and fat, 4 oz.	80
Beef, roasted, lean only, 4 oz.	80
Chicken, breast, roasted, 1/2 breast	80
Ham, sliced, 2 slices	30
Lamb chop, broiled, 4 oz.	95
Turkey, roasted, 4 oz.	60
Meats: Fish, Shellfish	
Cod, baked, 1 fillet, 6 oz.	85
Crab, blue, cooked, 3oz.	85
Tuna, light meat, canned, 3 oz.	25
Mussels, 6	120
Salmon, broiled, 5 oz.	110
Shrimp, boiled, 16, 3 oz. flesh	165

Label Glossary

Walk into any grocery store and you may find yourself seduced by food labels with bright proclamations of "extra lean" or "low in saturated fat." Here's the skinny on what those health claims really mean:

Calorie Free—fewer than 5 calories per serving

Cholesterol Free—less than 2 milligrams of cholesterol and 2 grams (or less) of saturated fat per serving

Low Cholesterol—20 milligrams of cholesterol (or less) per serving and 2 grams of saturated fat (or less) per serving

Reduced Cholesterol—at least 25 percent less cholesterol than the regular version and 2 grams (or less) of saturated fat per serving

Lean—less than 10 grams of fat, 4.5 grams of saturated fat, and no more than 95 milligrams of cholesterol per 3 oz. serving

Extra-Lean—less than 5 grams of fat, 2 grams of saturated fat, and 95 milligrams of cholesterol per 3 oz. serving.

Light (Lite)—1/3 fewer calories or no more than 1/2 the fat of the regular version; or no more than 1/2 the sodium of the higher-sodium version

Fat Free—less than 0.5 grams of fat per serving

Low Fat—3 grams of fat (or less) per serving

Reduced or Less Fat—at least 25 percent less fat per serving than the regular version

Low in Saturated Fat—1 gram of saturated fat (or less) per serving and not more than 15 percent of calories from saturated fatty acids

Sugar Free—less than 0.5 grams of sugar per serving

14

How Fats Get Carried Away

Your digestive system is a marvel of nature. Every day a spectacular arrangement of pipes and funnels work in perfect harmony to usher food through your body and distribute nutrients where they are needed. This complicated system motors along tirelessly without any conscious thought from you. You could say miracles are happening every day right under your nose!

Down in the Mouth

A small amount of fat-splitting enzyme called lingual lipase is produced in your mouth. When you swallow fats and they pass into your stomach, this enzyme begins splitting off one fatty acid from triglycerides. Virtually no other breakdown of fats occurs until fat reaches your small intestine, where bile salts act as detergents and break the fats into small droplets. Lipases then split the fats into a mixture of free fatty acids, monoglycerides, and diglycerides. Bile acids and phospholipids act as detergents and help the smaller particles of digested fats pass into the cells of the walls of your small intestine. The bile salts are left behind but almost all fat is absorbed.

Within the cells further splitting of fats occurs. Then the fatty acids reform into new triglycerides. These are combined with proteins and incorporated into lipoproteins called chylomicrons, which pass into the thoracic duct in the neck and then into the bloodstream. Short-chain fatty acids and glycerol do not take this route but pass directly into the portal vein and go straight to your liver. Chylomicrons are important to transport triglycerides, cholesterol, and fat-soluble vitamins from the wall of your intestine to other parts of your body, where they can be used or stored. The core of the chylomicron particle contains triglycerides and the surface carries phospholipids, cholesterol, and compounds called apoproteins.

Cholesterol

Fats don't dissolve in water, so for transport in the blood they are combined with proteins. If they were not, they would float on top of your blood, just like cream does in milk that has not been homogenized. In combination, proteins and fats are called lipoproteins, and, in this form, fats can travel in your blood. Depending on how closely the lipoproteins are packed together, they are called:

- very low-density lipoproteins, or VLDL
- intermediate-density lipoproteins, or IDL
- lowdensity lipoproteins, or LDL
- highdensity lipoproteins, or HDL

Very Low-Density Lipoproteins

VLDLs consist of a little over 50 percent triglycerides plus some phospholipids and cholesterol. They are formed in your liver, either from triglycerides made from sugars consumed in a meal or snack, or between meals from fats that have been mobilized from stored fat deposits in the body. VLDLs take triglycerides to your body's tissues, where they are used for energy or kept in storage. At this stage, the cholesterol component dominates the VLDL.

Intermediate-Density Lipoproteins

Once the cholesterol component prevails, the VLDL increases in density to become an IDL, which, in turn, loses some of its fats and becomes a low-density lipoprotein.

Low-Density Lipoproteins

The major type of fat in LDL is cholesterol. Some of this is deposited in your peripheral tissues and into your arteries, where it can build up into deposits called plaque. The level of LDL in your blood is strongly correlated with coronary heart disease, hence its moniker "bad cholesterol."

High-Density Lipoproteins

HDL particles have about 45 percent of their fat as phospholipids and can pick up cholesterol from your peripheral tissues, forming a compound called HDL3. This in turn picks up more cholesterol as well as some phospholipids and proteins from VLDL to form HDL2. Once HDL2 gets to your liver, it is broken down and the cholesterol is excreted or used for making bile and hormones. It is HDL's scavengerlike activities that have earned it a reputation as the "good cholesterol." A high level of HDL reduces the risk of coronary heart disease.

Lipoprotein(a)

Lp(a) is another lipoprotein that increase your risk of cardiovascular disease. It is a genetic factor and high levels in your blood can double the risk of heart attack in men before age fifty-five. There is some evidence that trans-fatty acids in some margarines and processed fats can increase Lp(a) levels and red wine can decrease it.

15

TRANS-FATTY ACIDS

As mentioned earlier, the process of hydrogenation involves changing liquid vegetable fats and oils into solid or spreadable fats. While it makes the fats more stable, it also alters their chemical structures, creating a trans-fatty acid that is an enemy of your heart, affecting your body in much the same way as a saturated fat.

Research Results

Interestingly, vegetable fats were meant to be a healthful alternative to saturated animal fats. The attention to trans-fatty acids increased when medical researchers noted in several studies that a trans-fatty acid called elaidic acid formed during hydrogation of vegetable oils to produce a solid product, reduced levels of "good" cholesterol in the blood, and raised levels of "bad" cholesterol in the study participants. It can also increase levels of Lp(a), which in turn increases the risk of coronary heart disease.

> One major study of over 85,000 nurses found that those who had consumed plenty of foods high in elaidic acid (mainly margarine) had a 50 percent greater risk of coronary heart disease than those who ate less margarine.

Another major study did not support such findings. Researchers took samples of body fat from men who had already had a heart attack and also from control subjects. They collected samples from men from ten countries and analyzed them to see if those who had suffered a heart attack had more trans-fatty acids in their body fat than those who had remained healthy. They found no significant difference between the two groups, although this may have been due to their inability to distinguish between trans-fatty acids that occur naturally and the elaidic acid produced by partial hydrogenation of oils. Levels of trans fats differed greatly between countries. The researchers did not rule out the possibility of a greater effect of trans fats on people in countries where the intake is high. Both groups from Spain had low levels of trans fats in their body fat, probably because their major dietary fat is olive oil, not margarine or processed fats. Spain has a very low level of coronary heart disease. Medical research is difficult at the best of times, but research on dietary factors is especially so. One researcher has suggested that elaidic acid may be harmful only when a person is consuming too many calories. Enough studies have now suggested that elaidic acid is undesirable and the food industry should exclude it from processed foods. This fat is not necessary, and there are many better though not necessarily cheaper ways to produce solid fats if they are indispensible for some processed foods.

It's worth noting that the naturally occurring trans-fatty acids in meat and dairy products function differently in your body and so are not of concern. (These foods have a high content of saturated fatty acids that can cause other problems.)

You can find high levels of the trans fat, elaidic acid, and trans-fatty acids in shortening used for doughnuts, pies, hamburger rolls, and other processed foods. Elaidic acid is commonly used by the food industry because it is an inexpensive way to increase the shelf life of processed foods. In areas of

India and Pakistan, a partly hydrogenated vegetable oil called vanaspathi is used. It contains very high levels of elaidic acid. The *British Medical Journal* reported that people living in areas where this type of fat is consumed have a high level of coronary heart disease.

Into the Fire

Margarines can be produced with minimal quantities of elaidic acid, but many manufacturers find themselves at a crossroad. They can either make products containing elaidic acid, the undesirable trans-fatty acid, or they can avoid it by increasing the level of saturated fatty acids—another undesirable feature.

Some margarine manufacturers have taken heed of the potentially adverse effects of this trans fat and are making their products with minimal quantities. Others believe the hazards have been overstated and they continue to sell polyunsaturated or monounsaturated margarines containing up to 15 percent of elaidic acid.

> Currently the Food and Drug Administration is considering the inclusion of trans-fatty acid content on food labels.

The problem for the margarine manufacturers is how to rank fatty acids according to which are the most undesirable. The problem for the consumer lies in knowing which is the best of a bad lot. The best solution may be to skip yellow fat spreads as much as possible.

Of even greater concern is the trend toward using hardened canola and cottonseed oils in processed foods. These products can have up to 45 percent trans fats, present as elaidic acid. More and more are being used in French fries and other foods with labels claiming that they have been prepared with canola oil, without mentioning that the canola oil has first been hardened and is contributing trans fats. Health-conscious consumers often choose these products, believing them to be superior. Better labeling seems imperative to help people who would prefer to avoid trans fats. Until we get it, frying with olive oil would be the healthiest choice.

Hydrogenated soybean oil used in baking and frying has 30 to 50 percent trans-fatty acids. Margarines may have 23 percent trans fats. Our estimated intake of trans-fatty acids is 8 to 12 grams, although some people may easily consume up to 40 grams a day. In the Netherlands, where fish and vegetable oils are commonly hydrogenated, daily consumption is estimated as 17 grams.

Some fast food restaurants upset at criticism of their widespread use of saturated fats have opted for frying in hydrogenated oil instead. This is truly a case of jumping out of the frying pan into the fire.

16

YOUR FOOD
HAS CHARACTER

Foods contain a mixture of types of fats, but particular foods are usually described by the dominant type of fatty acid. For example, olive oil is described as "monounsaturated" because the major portion (about 72 percent) of its fat is in the form of oleic acid, a monounsaturated fatty acid. Olive oil, however, also contains some saturated and some polyunsaturated fatty acids. When it is converted into an olive oil–based margarine, it can also gain some trans-fatty acids as a result of the processing.

Melting Points

The dominant type of fatty acid present in a fat influences the melting point. The molecular structure of most unsaturated fats is kinked and bent, which makes it difficult for the carbon chains of fatty acids to join together and lowers their melting point. Saturated or trans fats have a higher melting point because their carbon atoms occur close together in a straight line, in crystalline structures that do not melt easily.

In the kitchen you can get a good idea of which fatty acids predominate in foods by the solidity of the fat. Butter goes hard in the refrigerator because it has a high content of saturated fat. Adding some oil, as in dairy blend products, softens it because there is more unsaturated fat present. Beef fat is solid with its high percentage of saturated fatty acids, and lamb fat is so saturated that it will harden at room temperature. Chicken and pork fat, by contrast, stay fairly soft even in the refrigerator. The fat in ocean trout or salmon is always soft because it is unsaturated. Most fish have this kind of fat so they won't freeze in their cold-water environment. Oils are liquid because of their high content of unsaturated fatty acids. The table below tells you which fatty acids dominate some common foods.

Food	Type of fat (in grams)		
	Saturated	Monounsaturated	Polyunsaturated
Dairy Products			
Milk, whole, 1 cup	5	2	0
Milk, 2 % fat, 1 cup	3	1	0
Milk, 1 % fat, 1 cup	2	1	0
Milk, skim, 1 cup	0	0	0
Milk, goat's, 1 cup	7	3	<1
Milk, soy, 1 cup	1	1	3
Cream, half-and-half, 1 tbs.	1	1	0
Cheese, blue, 1 oz.	5	2	<1
Cheese, brie, 1 oz.	5	2	<1
Cheese, cheddar, 1 oz.	6	3	<1
Cheese, cottage, 2% fat, 1 cup	3	1	0
Cheese, cream, 2 tbs.	6	3	<1
Cheese, feta, 1 oz.	4	1	0
Cheese, mozzarella, shredded, 1/2 cup	7	4	0
Cheese, parmesan, 2 tbsp.	2	1	0
Cheese, ricotta, part skim, 1/2 cup	6	3	<1
Yogurt, low-fat, plain, 8 oz.	5	2	0
Ice cream, vanilla, 1 cup	9	4	<1
Ice cream, extra rich, vanilla, 1 cup	15	7	1
Eggs			
Egg, white, 1	0	0	0
Egg, yolk, 1	2	2	1
Egg, boiled or poached, 1	2	2	1
Eggs, scrambled, 2	4	6	3

Food	Type of fat (in grams)		
	Saturated	Monounsaturated	Polyunsaturated
Meats: Beef, Lamb, Pork			
Beef, roast, 4 oz.	4	4	1
Beef, pot roast, lean, 4 oz.	9	10	1
Beef, ground, lean, broiled, 4 oz.			
Beef, sirloin, broiled, 11 oz.	17	19	2
Lamb, chop, broiled, 4 oz.	4	4	1
Pork, bacon, 3 pc.	3	5	1
Pork, ham, roasted, 4 oz.	6	7	2
Pork, chop, broiled, 3 oz. with bone	4	5	1
Meats: Fish and Shellfish			
Fish, cod, baked, 1 fillet, 6 oz.	<1	<1	1
Fish, flounder, baked, 1 fillet, 6 oz.	<1	<1	1
Fish, halibut, baked, 1/2 fillet, 5 oz.	<1	1	2
Fish, salmon, baked, 1/2 fillet, 5 oz.	2	4	5
Fish, trout, baked, 6 oz.	2	5	2
Fish, tuna, canned, in brine, 3 oz.	<1	<1	1
Fish, tuna, canned, oil-packed, 3 oz.	1	3	3
Lobster meat, steamed, 1 cup	0	0	<1
Oysters, Pacific, simmered, 5	1	1	2
Shrimp, boiled, 16, 3 oz. flesh	0	0	1
Meats: Poultry			
Chicken, breast, 1/2 average, roasted	2	3	2
Chicken, drumstick, battered, fried, 1	3	5	3
Turkey, dark meat, roasted, 4 oz.	2	2	2
Turkey, light meat, roasted, 4 oz.	1	1	1
Nuts			
Almonds, roasted, 2 oz.	2	19	7
Brazil, 2 oz.	9	13	14
Cashew, dry roasted, 2 oz.	4	15	4
Coconut, fresh, 1 piece, 1 1/2 oz.	13	1	0
Coconut, desiccated, 1 tbs.	5	0	0
Hazelnuts, 2 oz.	2	26	5

Food	Type of fat (in grams)		
	Saturated	Monounsaturated	Polyunsaturated
Macadamia, roasted, 2 oz.	7	33	1
Peanuts, roasted, 2 oz.	4	14	9
Peanut butter, 2 tbs.	3	8	4
Pecans, 2 oz.	4	25	12
Pistachio, shelled, roasted, 2 oz.	3	14	8
Pumpkin seeds, roasted, 2 oz.	2	3	5
Sesame seeds, dry, 1 tbs.	<1	2	2
Sunflower seeds, 2 oz.	3	5	19
Tahini paste, 1 tbs.	1	3	4
Walnuts, 2 oz.	3	5	26
Oils			
Canola, 1 tbs.	1	9	4
Corn or maize, 1 tbs.	2	3	8
Olive, 1 tbs.	2	10	1
Peanut, 1 tbs.	2	6	4
Safflower, regular, 1 tbs.	1	2	10
Safflower, high oleic, 1 tbs.	1	10	2
Soybean, 1 tbs.	2	3	8
Sunflower, 1 tbs.	1	3	9
Fats			
Butter, 1 tbs.	7	3	<1
Margarine, hard, 1 tbs.	2	5	4
Margarine, soft, 1 tbs.	2	4	5
Lard, 1 tbs.	5	6	1
Chicken fat, 1 tbs.	4	6	3
Chocolate, milk, 1 1/2 oz. bar	8	4	0
Chocolate, sweet, dark, 1 1/2 oz. bar	8	5	0
Mayonnaise, 1 tbs.	1	1	3

Margarine

You might be surprised to know that polyunsaturated and monounsaturated margarines are a major source of saturated fats. The oils they are made from usually contain quite low contents of saturated fatty acids. To turn these oils into more spreadable products, they are combined with fats high in saturated or trans-fatty acids. Some have a bit of both. If margarines did not have some saturated or trans fats, they would still be oils. In making poly- and monounsaturated margarines, unsaturated oils are combined with enough saturated fats or trans-fatty acids to form a spread. It is not possible to have a spreadable fat without one or another of these less desirable components. Even if the major type of fat present is unsaturated, regular margarines, like butter, consist of 80 percent fat, so the number of grams of saturated fat in an average serving is high. For example, a tablespoon of poly or monounsaturated margarine has almost a teaspoon of saturated and trans fat (as well as its other fats) whereas the much-maligned egg has less than half a teaspoon of saturated fat. Many people avoid eggs but happily use margarine on toast, in mashed potato, for frying, and in cooking.

17

THE OXIDATION OF FATS

Fats become rancid, or smell a bit "off," when oxygen attacks their fatty acid chain in a process known as oxidation. Some types of fatty acids oxidize more rapidly than others.

The Omegas

Omega 3 Fatty Acids

Omega 3 fatty acids, such as those found in flaxseed oil or fish, are the least stable and the most likely to oxidize if exposed to oxygen in the air. That is why fish does not keep long and why fish that isn't fresh can be picked by its odor. It is also a major reason why it is difficult to enjoy the benefits of flaxseed oil.

Canola oil also contains some omega 3 fatty acids that oxidize easily.

> If you have ever tried deep-frying with canola, or even shallow-frying for more than a minute or two, you may have noticed a fishy smell. It comes from the breakdown of the omega 3 fatty acid: alpha-linolenic acid.

The richest source of alpha-linolenic acid is flaxseed (also known as linseed) oil. It is so unstable that it can be kept only for a short time, and then only if it is cold and in a brown bottle away from light. Once attacked by oxygen, the breakdown of its fatty acids is inevitable. For this reason it is difficult to use it for cooking. Keeping flaxseeds inside their protective coating in a cool place is the best way to prevent the fats from becoming rancid.

Omega 6 Fatty Acids

Omega 6 fatty acids found in polyunsaturated oils also oxidize readily during storage and cooking, and also in cell membranes in your body. A single use in deep-frying breaks down some of the fats in polyunsaturated oils through a process known as hydro-peroxidation. The compounds formed then destroy the oil's antioxidants so that it oxidizes rapidly. Polyunsaturated oils, like corn, safflower, and sesame, should only ever be used once. Any leftovers after frying should be thrown out. Olive oil, by contrast, has such high levels of naturally occurring antioxidants as well as mainly monounsaturated fat that it can be used many times before any undesirable fatty acids form. In practice this more than compensates for its initial high price.

Once polyunsaturated fats take up residence in your cell membranes or as part of low-density lipoproteins in your arteries, the requirement for antioxidants also increases.

> **The recommended daily intake of vitamin E, one of the antioxidant vitamins, is directly related to the intake of polyunsaturated fatty acids.**

While some of these fats are also good sources of vitamin E, they can be destroyed by cooking or some types of processing. Many commercial oils are extracted using a chemical solvent, which must then be removed, but this means that many of the original protective substances are also removed. Again, olive oil has an advantage, as it is produced by cold pressing. Only olive oil marked "pomace oil" is extracted with a chemical solvent.

Saturated Fatty Acids

Very short-chain saturated fatty acids found in butter and dairy products also oxidize easily and give rise to the slightly "off" flavor in butter that is no longer fresh. The fats from goat's and sheep milk also oxidize readily, and this is presented as a "plus" because it contributes to the distinctive flavor of the cheeses made from these milks.

Rancidity

The oxidation of fats is commonly called rancidity. It is undesirable from a gastronomic viewpoint and also harmful for health because oxidized fatty acids can damage arteries. Antioxidants help prevent oxidation. Most margarines and some oils and cooking fats have an antioxidant added to prevent rancidity, because many of their natural antioxidants are destroyed by processing.

Makers of processed and fast foods use vegetable oils that have been converted into saturated fats or trans-fatty acids because they are less likely to oxidize and therefore have a longer shelf life than that of the unsaturated oils in their original forms.

PART III

Food and Your Health

Throughout the history of the world, most people thought fat was good. In the quantities that many ate, it probably was. There is now a common misconception spreading rapidly throughout developed countries that fat is undesirable, but the effects of fat on your health depend primarily on the quantity and type of fats you eat. Some fatty acids are essential, and a certain amount of fat is important at all ages. Fat is vital for growth and survival during infancy. In most Western countries, however, the intake of *saturated* fats has become excessive and is related to many health problems.

18

A HEALTHY HEAD START

Infants have a greater need for fat than any other age group. For the first few days of life a newborn baby gets colostrum from its mother's breasts. Colostrum is high in protein and rich in compounds that give the baby immunity to infection. There is less fat in colostrum than in mature breast milk, but more than twice as much cholesterol. Colostrum is also rich in fat-soluble vitamins—about three times the level present in mature breast milk. At all ages, fat-soluble vitamins need dietary fat for their absorption.

As the colostrum gives way to transitional milk, the fat content rises and the cholesterol falls slightly. When mature milk comes in on about the third or fourth day after giving birth, it has even more fat. The breastfed infant continues to get more than half its calories from fat, and this level is vitally important to provide babies with a package of concentrated energy for fast growth. The American Academy of Pediatrics recommends breastfeeding for six to twelve months, so ideally, breastfeeding should continue until your baby is one year old. Solid foods can commence when the baby is six months old.

For the first year, the high fat content and other important nutrients of milk play a major role in the infant's growth.

Infant mortality rates are lower for breastfed babies than bottle-fed in third world countries.

Breast Is Best

Breast milk is a beautiful, life-giving liquid that has a nutritional code researchers have been puzzling over for years. It's a very complex substance, with over 50 percent of its calories coming from fat. There is no generally accepted theory about why so much of the fat in breast milk is saturated or why its cholesterol level is so high. Some researchers have suggested that when the diet provides ready-made cholesterol, the infant's liver will not need to make its own supplies and will be more able to turn off its cholesterol-synthesis mechanism when it is not needed in later life.

Others think it is simply that infants need high levels of cholesterol to produce plenty of the bile acids required for digesting the high-fat diet that is essential for their rapid growth. Infant formulas fall short of providing the pure nutritional value of breast milk, although manufacturers are striving to make them closer to breast milk.

Some infant formulas now contain some added omega 3 fatty acids, but they still do not match the complexity and type of fatty acids found in breast milk.

Breast milk has a relatively high level of polyunsaturated omega 3 fatty acids, especially DHA (docosahexaenoic acid). It is not possible to research all of DHA's effects on the brain, but studies show that breastfed babies have sharper vision than those fed on formula milks, probably for at least their first six months. The effect is most pronounced in babies born prematurely.

A number of careful studies have shown that children who were breastfed as babies have higher IQs than children fed formula. Researchers who have come up with statistics to prove this have tried to account for the fact that mothers who breastfeed have higher education levels, but it is difficult to isolate such factors completely. However, with eight out of ten studies showing positive results, this is yet another reason to encourage breastfeeding.

The pattern of fatty acids in breast milk should be a guide for manufacturers of infant formulas. Most aim to match the natural product and many have been trying to find a way to introduce more omega 3 fatty acids into infant formulas. They cannot simply add DHA, because it is an unstable molecule and oxidizes readily to form harmful compounds. Alpha-linolenic acid, a potential building block for DHA, is also unstable, but some manufacturers have overcome technical difficulties and incorporated it into some of their products.

19

NUTRITION DURING CHILDHOOD AND ADOLESCENCE

The appetites of children are directly related to their growth. One day they shun all food set before them and the next they seem to devour everything in their paths. Growth spurts and times of extra physical activity mean children's bodies require extra nutrition and the right level of calories to keep up with their needs.

Fat Grows Up

Breast milk provides enough fat to support the growth of babies. As children grow and are weaned, they still need calories from fat, and after twelve months of age, cow's milk is a useful source. The fat in milk is important for the absorption of vitamins A, D, E, and K. Children should have regular milk rather than low-fat milk, at least for their first few years. There is no problem in using low-fat milk in puddings or other occasional foods.

As in infancy, children do not need lots of obviously fatty foods with poor nutrient levels. Instead, they should get their fat from products such as eggs, lean meat or poultry, cereals, peanut (or other nut) butter, milk, cheese, and yogurt, all of which supply nutrients important for growth and activity. A scrape of butter or margarine on toast is unlikely to cause problems, although it is not necessary.

High-fat extras such as potato chips, chocolate, cakes, and fast foods have no essential purpose and should be omitted or used only as occasional extras. Lots of us do not see any problem with children eating a lot of these junk foods with high levels of fat, assuming that children are active enough to burn them up. But we've overlooked the dental hazards of sweet fatty foods.

In days gone by, when children walked long distances and helped with heavy household tasks, some junk foods may not have been such a problem. Somewhat ironically, few such foods were available then.

> **These days, however, one in four American children is overweight or obese—double the incidence 25 years ago. Ten percent of adolescents between the ages of 12 and 19 have cholesterol levels over 200 mg/dl. The problem of child obesity is also increasing in Japan and other countries as they increase their consumption of fatty junk foods.**

There is no doubt that part of the blame for excess weight lies with decreasing physical activity that comes from children playing computer games and watching television instead of playing outside, being driven to school instead of walking, and having few energy-consuming household tasks assigned to them. But some blame for the high level of excess weight in children must also go to the food they eat. Years ago children ate a good deal of fruit, but today they are more likely to eat chips and other fatty snack foods. Chocolates, doughnuts, fast foods, and fried foods that were once reserved for special occasions have now become everyday fare. A diet high in such fatty foods quickly leads to an expanding group of overweight kids.

20

FATS AND YOUR HEART: WHAT RESEARCH TELLS US

Thanks to huge leaps in medical research today, our average life span far exceeds that of generations that lived before us. Many of the diseases that devastated our ancestors were infectious, such as influenza, tuberculosis, scarlet fever, and smallpox. Today we are able to identify offending micro-organisms and prevent illnesses that would have caused irreparable damage to our bodies not too long ago. Now modern technologies are taxed with preventing and treating chronic conditions caused partly by our genes but mostly by our environment and our lifestyle. One of those diseases is heart disease, the leading single cause of death among Americans. High levels of saturated fats in our diets almost certainly deserve some condemnation for their role in various types of heart disease.

The Smoking Gun

Until the 1950s, most nutrition researchers thought the key to good health was to have plenty of food, especially food rich in animal protein. This was an understandable viewpoint, as up to that time most nutrition-related health problems were due to a lack of some nutrient, or a general lack of food. Those in countries blessed with a rich supply of food, including high-fat meats and dairy products, appeared to have few problems, except among the poor who could not afford enough to eat.

During the 1950s, coronary heart disease reached almost epidemic proportions in wealthy countries, especially among middle-aged men. Researchers began to look for reasons. They soon discovered the link with cigarette smoking, and in the 1960s many major health organizations began public programs to educate us on the adverse effects of smoking. Since then, deaths from heart disease have steadily dropped. They continue to decline as research and technology develop new medications that protect the heart and extend our lives.

A World of Good

In the 1950s a group of researchers led by Dr. Ancel Keys coordinated a now-famous study known as the Seven Countries Study in which they looked at deaths from coronary heart disease and dietary patterns in eighteen populations in seven different countries.

Keys and his coworkers found that the total *amount* of fat that people ate had no relationship to coronary heart disease, but the *type* of fat was highly relevant.

People in countries such as Greece ate the most fat but had the least heart disease. Almost all the fat came from olive oil and nuts, with some from cheese and yogurt.

Mediterranean populations were not vegetarian but they ate little meat, and cakes, pastries, and other such goodies were eaten only for feasts and special occasions. Vegetables made flavorful with herbs, garlic, lemon, and olive oil featured strongly in their diets, along with fish, bread, other grain products, and a moderate, regular intake of red wine.

At the other end of the spectrum, people in Finland had the highest rate of heart disease. They also ate a lot of fat, but it came mainly from meat, butter, milk, and processed fats. Their vegetable consumption was low and they drank little red wine.

The total amount of fat consumed did not significantly differ between the diets of Finland and Greece, but the types of fats did. The Finnish diet, and that of populations with similarly high levels of heart disease, was dominated by saturated fat. These fats had only a minor role in the diet of all countries with low rates of heart disease.

The Japanese populations studied also had low levels of coronary heart disease but high levels of high blood pressure and stroke. Their diet was low in all fats, including saturated fats. Vegetables, fish, and rice were dominant foods. Their salt intake from soy sauce and salted fish was high and directly related to blood pressure and stroke.

> In spite of the importance and great publicity given to the Seven Countries Study, one of their essential findings was overlooked for many years. In their rush to condemn saturated fats such as butter and find an alternative, researchers and the food industry ignored the types of fats, and other foods, that Mediterranean people were eating.

The Move to Polyunsaturated Fats

Few dietary changes are free of bias, and most recommendations are pushed by someone who stands to make a profit from them. In this case, the oil seed industry saw a splendid opportunity to introduce a new range of highly profitable products—polyunsaturated oils and margarines. Advertisers made the most of the research findings that saturated fats were undesirable and that an alternative to a highly saturated product such as butter was highly preferable. They vigorously promoted polyunsaturated margarines along with safflower, sunflower, corn, and soybean oils, and health authorities supported these products at the time.

Research studies were carried out to support these assumptions, but these had an artificiality that distorted the results. Subjects were given experimental liquid diets containing different types of fats, and their blood cholesterol levels were measured. When these diets contained a lot of saturated fats, cholesterol levels rose. With large quantities of polyunsaturated fats, the levels fell. When given monounsaturated fats similar to those found in olive oil, their blood cholesterol levels did not change significantly. At this stage saturated fats were damned, polyunsaturated fats were praised, and monounsaturates were largely ignored.

> **Researchers overlooked the observation that people in Mediterranean countries who ate large quantities of monounsaturated fats in the form of olive oil had relatively low blood cholesterol levels, and at the time the lowest rate of coronary heart disease in the world.**

For the next thirty years researchers and health authorities concentrated on polyunsaturated fats and referred to P:S ratios (polyunsaturated to saturated). They ignored monounsaturated fats, even though they make up the bulk of fatty acids in many diets. It is not clear that the P:S ratio ever did more than simply indicate the quantity of polyunsaturated oils and margarine being consumed, but the ratio is still quoted. Its continued appeal demonstrates how usage tends to create status that persists long after usefulness has ended.

More than thirty years ago some researchers also showed that different saturated fatty acids did not have equal effects in raising serum cholesterol.

> **The candy industry picked up the fact that stearic acid, a saturated fatty acid that does *not* raise cholesterol, was present in chocolate. They did not give equal publicity to the fact that chocolate is also high in palmitic acid, which *does* raise blood cholesterol.**

Nor did they publicize the fact that stearic acid may cause blood platelets to stick together, increasing the chances of blood clots forming. This is an example of how research into fatty acids can be used to suit the purposes of a particular group with a product to sell.

In practice, most foods that are high in saturated fat contain a mixture of these fats rather than just one, and cutting back on all foods rich in saturated fats is the easiest way to reduce the less desirable saturated fatty acids. This is an example of how messages about diet and heart disease can be oversimplified so that they convey something other than the full truth. Scientific results are filtered through researchers and health authorities, some of whom may feel the facts are too complex for the public to understand. Still other researchers can become carried away with the results of test-tube meals and ignore the importance of the total diet.

The Move to Monounsaturated Fats

The advice to everyone to increase polyunsaturated fats seemed strange, especially in light of the fact that no human population had ever consumed such large quantities of these fats.

Polyunsaturated fats started their fall from grace during the 1970s and 1980s when medical researchers realized the importance of distinguishing between LDL cholesterol, which increases the risk of heart disease (the so-called "bad" cholesterol), and HDL cholesterol ("good" cholesterol), which reduces the risk. Once again they examined the effects of different classes of dietary fats given to volunteers.

> Saturated fats increased both types of blood cholesterol, although their effect on the "good" HDL type was small compared with their effect in raising "bad" LDL cholesterol.

Polyunsaturated fats given in high quantity turned out to lower both "good" and "bad" cholesterol levels—hence their assumed potency when only the total levels were being measured.

Monounsaturated fats, on the other hand, lowered "bad" cholesterol and seemed to have some potential to raise the "good" type, or at least favorably alter the ratio of "good" and "bad" cholesterol.

The conclusion at this stage was that saturated fats were still bad, and that polyunsaturates were undesirable in large doses but essential in small quantities. Researchers began to sing the praises of monounsaturated fats and manufacturers looked at ways of producing more of them.

Oxidization

The next stage in this saga of unfolding scientific research has occurred over the past ten to twenty years. The "bad" LDL cholesterol turns out to be a true villain only when it oxidizes. Polyunsaturated fats oxidize more readily than the more stable monounsaturates, mainly because the polyunsaturates have less stable double bonds in their molecules. This is why oils with a high content of polyunsaturated fat go rancid quickly in your kitchen. It occurs in the frying pan, especially if a polyunsaturated oil is used more than once. Oxidation can also occur in your arteries, where free-radical molecules produced as body tissues age attack polyunsaturated fats carried in low-density lipoproteins. Once these fats are degraded by the oxidation reaction, they are taken up into foam cells and also form substances that increase the chances of your blood cells clumping together to form a clot. Oxidized fats lead to the formation of inflammatory substances too, and also interfere with the ability of the cells lining the artery to relax.

This oxidation reaction does not occur readily with saturated fatty acids and is slow with monounsaturated fatty acids. However, a diet high in refined polyunsaturates can present a greater risk for atherosclerosis, unless more antioxidants are also supplied to prevent oxidation.

> In nature, most polyunsaturated fats occur with plenty of antioxidants. When they are refined, however, many of the protective accompaniments are lost.

Advice through the Years

It is worthwhile looking at the history of dietary recommendations for coronary heart disease because they illustrate how greater knowledge can alter the emphasis in dietary advice. The early studies focused on the effects of diet on total serum cholesterol, until it became known that the type of cholesterol that increases the risk of coronary heart disease is carried in low-density lipoproteins (LDL). Cholesterol in high-density lipoproteins (HDL) decreases the risk of coronary heart disease. The change of emphasis does not invalidate the conclusions drawn from the initial studies. It just means that they did not look at the whole picture. The nature of the intricate work being done by most researchers means that many will continue to attach great importance to the single issue they are studying.

Buyer Beware

Buying habits can be very telling when it comes to gauging how nutritional recommendations are being received. When told that polyunsaturated margarine was good for us, we bought it. The fact that it was easily spreadable and cheaper than butter probably helped sales, but it was the health message that won us over to a product we had rejected, because of its taste, before the mid-1970s. Now that we are hearing health messages about monounsaturated fats, many of us are switching to monounsaturated margarine and buying and enjoying olive oil. Sales of olive oil have increased dramatically over the past couple of years—formerly, only small bottles of it were sold in pharmacies or the therapeutic goods section of the supermarket, but olive oil now dominates the oil section. Where confusion does arise, it could be due to conflicting sales pitches from those who are marketing foods rich in mono- or polyunsaturates.

Saturated fats are still damned—and there is no evidence to support reinstating them to any positive health status—but monounsaturates have at last been accepted.

> **Unfortunately, some people have taken the antifat message to heart so much that the compulsion to condemn all fats comes pretty easily. This may be unwise.**

When people eat very little fat of any kind, their blood levels of LDL cholesterol are low. They produce very little LDL cholesterol and their bodies break down very little. A moderate intake of saturated fats and a high intake of monounsaturated fats, as consumed in Mediterranean countries, may help the body break down some LDL cholesterol. By contrast, a high intake of saturated fats and a low consumption of monounsaturates, as occurs in parts of northern Europe, produces lots of LDL cholesterol and very little is broken down.

LDL cholesterol production is due to eating a lot of saturated fat. The breakdown of LDL cholesterol is greater with a higher intake of monounsaturated fatty acids, so these fats may protect us against the damaging effects of high blood cholesterol. Polyunsaturates have a lesser role in this respect.

Antioxidants

A relatively new player entered the arena when theories about oxidation became accepted. Antioxidants have been big news over the past twenty years—and antioxidant supplements are selling well. As their name suggests, antioxidants can prevent oxidation reactions. Foods contain literally thousands of antioxidants: vegetables, fruits, nuts, olive oil, red wine, and tea are the major sources. With the exception of tea, all these foods dominate the Mediterranean diets.

> **We could probably have saved fifty years of going around in a circle if we had taken note of what Mediterranean people ate and followed suit.**

We might also have taken up some of the obvious pleasures that Mediterranean people enjoy as they sit down with friends and family to their wonderfully tasty and healthy foods.

Olive Oil

We should learn from this that no single food is responsible for good health. Olive oil has mainly monounsaturated fats, which are now acknowledged as beneficial. But olive oil also contains dozens of potent antioxidants that may be equally beneficial. This point is still being ignored by those who produce and market other monounsaturated oils that lack olive oil's variety of antioxidants.

Canola Oil

There are advertisements carrying Mediterranean recipes that use highly processed canola oil, bred from rapeseeds to remove their harmful erucic acid, extracted with a solvent and containing one added antioxidant to replace those lost during processing. This product may well be a useful oil, but it has nothing to do with the virtues of the Mediterranean diet. Canola oil reduces LDL cholesterol levels nicely, but we simply do not know its other effects at this stage.

Perhaps its worst feature is that it has been processed to have no flavor—just when we are learning that many of the most potent antioxidants are found in the flavor components of foods.

Flaxseed Oil

Sometimes a little knowledge has been a dangerous thing. Flaxseeds are a valuable source of alpha-linolenic acid, an omega 3 fatty acid. In fact, flaxseeds are so rich in this highly unstable fatty acid that the oil goes rancid within hours or days of being squeezed from the seeds. (The short life span of its fatty acids is one reason flaxseed oil is used in paints.) Some researchers decided flaxseed oil could be used as a food if the plants were altered so that they had less of this easily oxidized fatty acid. The oil extracted from the seeds of this new plant was christened linola. Since then, however, we have discovered omega 3 fatty acids are the valuable part of flaxseeds. The new oil took a wrong turn, thanks to the incomplete knowledge of the time. Eating flaxseeds themselves solves some of the problems of oxidation. As long as they are kept in the fridge, the oil is protected within the seeds. Food manufacturers, however, see flaxseeds as much less attractive, since few people will consume such great quantities as they might with a margarine made from their oil. This is where commercial food interests and good nutrition are incompatible. Wise eating demands moderation; marketing wants ever-increasing consumption.

Sunflower Seed Oil

Plant geneticists have been busily changing sunflowers to decrease their usual polyunsaturated fatty acids and to increase their monounsaturated content. This is to give a more marketable ingredient for margarine now that there is widespread criticism of high intakes of polyunsaturated products. But is it necessary, or would it be better to eat some regular sunflower seeds and skip margarine altogether? Some polyunsaturated fatty acids are essential to the diet. Sunflower seeds have always been a well-balanced source, supplying plenty of antioxidants along with their polyunsaturated fatty acids. Will these still be present in the same proportions once the fatty acids are changed in the genetically modified monounsaturated sunflowers? The plant, after all, produces its antioxidants to match the needs of its fats.

Which Changes Are Best?

Research has been hampered by people trying to push particular products. Sales of antioxidant vitamins (A, C, and E) are at an all-time high: the advertisements imply that they will save you from cancer, heart disease, and arthritis. Most of the most potent antioxidants in foods have less familiar names, many of them difficult to pronounce, which will make it hard to market any of them as supplements. Such a move would also be absurd, since the fact that they exist in the thousands in a single fruit or vegetable may well be the major reason for their potency. For a list of antioxidant-rich foods, refer to Chapter 22.

Oversimplified messages in advertisements and on food labels can lead to changes that are not necessarily ideal, and may at best be compromises. You should always look at why certain products are being promoted and whether promotions convey the full message.

21

DO YOUR HEART GOOD

In 1908 scientists were studying the arteries of rabbits and found them clogged with fatty deposits that hindered blood flow. These rabbits weren't eating their preferred diet of carrots and lettuce, but rather a more "humanlike" diet of meat, whole milk, and eggs. That group of researchers were the first to identify the substance we commonly call cholesterol. Three years later a Dutch physician working in Java, Indonesia, discovered that the natives had lower rates of heart disease than Dutch colonists who were also living on the island. Dr. Cornelius de Langen hypothesized that the healthier hearts were due to low levels of blood cholesterol. He also noted that when Indonesians strayed from their typical diet of plant foods and ate lots of meat and dairy products, their risk for heart disease climbed. Unfortunately, these important findings were buried for four decades.

Eggs

The message that *cholesterol is harmful* is another example of a simple message that went wrong. You may be part of a large group of people who are unaware of distinctions between the cholesterol in foods and blood cholesterol. It's vital to know that one does not necessarily lead to another, and concentrating on food sources of cholesterol has led to some inappropriate changes and neglect of the real problem. For example, if you have high blood cholesterol, you may have cut eggs out of your diet. Over the years this has become a knee-jerk reaction.

> **The American Heart Association has approved eating up to 4 eggs a week when other dietary sources of cholesterol are limited.**

We are beginning to get the message that eggs are not "deviled." Since 1991 our consumption of eggs has been rising and will probably continue to rise as more and more of us accept eggs back into our fridge. For example, an egg has 5 grams of total fat and less than 2 grams of saturated fat. If it is replaced by a bowl of granola with 1 percent reduced-fat milk (which most people think is a healthy choice), the fat content in the "healthier" choice will range from 10–32 grams of total fat, including 2–7 grams of saturated fat (range depends on type of granola used).

You should also question whether some people may be disadvantaged by removing eggs from their diet. The *real* message to reduce blood cholesterol is to cut back on saturated fat. The once standard breakfast of bacon and fried eggs was high in fat and saturated fat, but its demise has turned an entire population off a nutritious food, which can also be easily incorporated into many low-fat, inexpensive meals. Many of us wanted a quick, easy meal, and would have once used eggs. We now have fast foods, most of which have a much higher content of fat.

> **Two eggs and toast have less than half the fat of a fast food hamburger.**

The desire for a simple message—*cholesterol is bad*—has led to confusion between dietary and blood cholesterol. A more complicated message might have conveyed a more accurate message.

Replacing Saturated Fats

In France, Spain, Greece, and southern Italy, people eat large quantities of cheese and yogurt, yet rates of coronary heart disease are low. It may be that other foods such as vegetables, olive oil, nuts, and red wine provide enough protection against the undesirable properties of the saturated fats in cheese and yogurt. It is also possible that when milk is fermented to make cheese and yogurt, alterations in either the arrangement of fatty acids on their triglyceride backbone or some aspect of the changes in proteins in the foods overrides the saturated fats. Or it may be that when the sheep and goats of the region graze on wild greens, their milk contains protective omega 3 fatty acids.

Such strong evidence should make you reconsider removing all sources of saturated fat from your diet. Instead, reduce the foods that are drenched in saturated fats, such as fast and fried foods, baked goods, pastries, butter, and sweets as the first step toward keeping your heart humming.

The two most likely contenders to replace excess saturated fat are starchy foods or monounsaturated fats. There are historical precedents and evidence supporting both courses of action.

> **The healthful diet that contributes to longevity in Japan has lots of rice to provide calories from its starchy carbohydrate, as well as vegetables, legumes, some nuts, fish and other seafoods, and fresh fruit. Other foods have traditionally been used only in small quantities.**

The healthful Mediterranean diets use monounsaturated fats as a major source of calories. They come mostly from olive oil, with nuts also an important source, along with other commonly eaten foods rich in protective antioxidants.

Are Americans a Bad Influence?

The debate about which is the best substitute for excess saturated fat is likely to go on for some time. Meanwhile, the traditional diets that have proved protection against coronary heart disease are disappearing in their places of origin as fast food companies and food manufacturers move in to increase their world market dominance, and as local people adopt American-style eating habits for convenience in their increasingly time-strapped lives.

We are already seeing increases in coronary heart disease and decreases in longevity in countries such as Greece, and similar effects are expected in Japan as risk factors increase with changing ways of life. In Lyon, France, people who had already had one heart attack were randomly assigned either to a Mediterranean-style diet or one based on low-fat recommendations from the American Heart Association. Blood cholesterol levels stayed much the same in each group, but there was a 70 percent reduction in deaths from heart attacks in the group given the Mediterranean diet. This dramatic reduction occurred without any significant reduction in blood cholesterol.

Gone Fishin'

Another similar trial that has successfully reduced deaths from heart attacks and other coronary events was conducted in Wales, where an increased fish intake was given credit, and in Norway, in which participants reduced saturated fat without increasing polyunsaturated fat and ate more fish, fruit, and vegetables.

These trials are important because none of them used a diet high in the kind of polyunsaturated fats heart associations contend can lower cholesterol levels. No intervention/prevention trial has ever found it successful in preventing coronary deaths.

A diet high in the kind of polyunsaturates found in margarine and many vegetable oils (linoleic acid) does reduce blood cholesterol and there is no doubt that this is important. But lowering total blood cholesterol is only one factor and by itself may not always be enough to decrease deaths from coronary heart disease and other causes.

The chief researcher in the Lyon study has shown that when linoleic acid is increased enough to reduce blood cholesterol, blood platelets may stick together more, increasing the risk of blood clots forming. Eating more fish will help prevent this.

The American Heart Association recommends eating two servings a week of fish, like tuna and salmon.

The authors of the Lyon Heart Study suggest that the protective effect of their dietary pattern may have been due to several factors:

1. monounsaturated fat (which oxidizes less rapidly than polyunsaturates)
2. more natural antioxidants (from fruits, vegetables, legumes, and wine)
3. or alpha-linolenic acid (usually present in Mediterranean diets as the green leafy vegetable known as purslane)

They also noted that since serum cholesterol levels were not significantly different in the experimental or control groups, but no sudden death occurred in the Mediterranean diet group (compared with many deaths in the control group), the protective effect of their diet may have been the reduction of changes in heart rhythm (arrhythmias), or the lower incidence of platelets clumping together. These factors are sometimes forgotten when so much emphasis is given to cholesterol. Several studies have shown that omega 3 fatty acids in fish oils reduce arrhythmias in rats and in humans. The Lyon Heart Study's use of the omega 3 alpha-linolenic acid and the Welsh and Norwegian trials support this.

A number of other studies using diets with a relatively
high content of fat derived largely from nuts (mainly
monounsaturated fat) reduced coronary heart disease
risk more than diets with less total fat but more polyunsaturated fat.

People with type 2 (non-insulin-dependent) diabetes have a
higher than average risk of coronary heart disease. Their diabetes
is controlled better if they adopt a diet with more monounsaturated fat compared with one that is low in fat and higher in carbohydrate.

The heart disease diet recommendations have also been
complicated by changing opinions about trans-fatty acids.
Once considered unimportant, the type of trans-fatty acids
present in the margarines and fats that are used in many
processed foods are at least as undesirable as saturated fatty
acids. These fats were discussed in greater detail in Chapter 15.

The Heart of the Matter

There is now such a body of scientific and medical literature on
the subject of diet and heart disease that you can find studies to
support many points of view, but not all those studies or points
of view are necessarily valid. More than ever, it is important to
view the subject overall, rather than isolating one aspect.

Some aspects of the links between diet and heart disease
have not changed. For example, for adults, it is still desirable to
reduce saturated fat. Previous recommendations to increase
consumption of polyunsaturated fats, however, no longer apply.
These fats are fine in moderation, but more is not better. If you
want to reduce your risk of coronary heart disease you should:

1. decrease saturated fats
2. select monounsaturated fats rather than take in a large
   amount of polyunsaturated fats

3. ensure an adequate intake of antioxidants
4. avoid high levels of trans-fatty acids
5. eat fish or other seafood twice a week

If the diets of healthy populations with low levels of coronary heart disease were explored more carefully, we could have adopted similar eating patterns decades ago. Asian, Mediterranean, and Middle Eastern diets naturally capture all the recommendations above.

22

DIETARY FAT AND CANCER

Cancer is the second leading cause of death in the United States. However, it is the number one cause of death for people between the ages of forty-five and sixty-four. Even more alarming is that many of those deaths could have been prevented with a change in lifestyle. However, according to the National Cancer Institute, the rates for new cancer cases are declining in the United States. Medical research is making incredible strides in treating cancer, so many people who are stricken have good reason to feel hopeful today.

Environmental factors are involved in many cancers, although the exact percentages attributable to factors such as cigarette smoking, diet, and contact with high levels of various chemical substances are debatable. Most experts agree that about a third of all cancers may be related to what we eat and drink.

The subject of diet and cancer is complex.

Some people assume that food additives are the major problem, but more evidence points to fat as the major culprit in a number of different types of cancers, particularly breast, colon, and prostate. A high-fat diet tends to be low in whole grains, fruits, and vegetables—foods that contain hundreds of factors that can protect us against many cancer-causing agents. A high-fat diet is also high in total energy and this has been shown in many animal studies to increase the risk of cancer.

It is strange that in countries with bountiful supplies of fruits and vegetables, the consumption of them is dropping.

Many people feel they don't have time to eat these healthful foods. Advertising makes fatty fast foods a tempting replacement. This results in a double whammy—too much fat and not enough protective food factors. It's not clear which is the more relevant to the increasing incidence of some cancers.

In the development of cancers, defective genes may increase vulnerability to disease. Not all defective genes result in cancer. Malignancy usually involves three stages:

1. initiation—the process whereby a defective gene reacts to an *initiator* (such as cigarette smoking or certain chemicals)
2. promotion—an element that causes the cells to become cancerous
3. progression—the process whereby the cancerous cells multiply to become a tumor

Diet may be involved in all stages. Foods may also offer protection against cancer, and what we eat and drink (or fail to eat) may give cells greater (or less) resistance to cancer-causing substances (carcinogens).

Cancer Sites

The subject of food and cancer is not simple. Carcinogens are sometimes present in foods or may be produced during the cooking or preservation of foods. Fat or other dietary substances may also initiate or promote changes in cells or activate carcinogens, while protective factors in foods may deactivate them.

There are many examples of how diet increases the risk of cancer. Epidemiological studies provide the first clues and research then tries to find the specific factors involved, including aspects of diet. They may differ according to the site of each cancer. For example:

Stomach cancer has been associated with a high salt intake.

This type of cancer is uncommon in the United States, but is very common in China, Japan, Korea, and other Asian countries, and is relatively common in parts of eastern Europe and Latin America. It is thought that high doses of sodium chloride from dried and salted foods rather than the total daily intake of sodium may damage the cells lining the stomach. A lack of fresh raw fruits and vegetables is also a factor because it deprives the cells of their essential protection.

Colon cancer is linked to a high-fat diet that may increase the production of bile acids. Once these acids have transported partly digested fats into the wall of the intestine, they pass to the large intestine (colon), where they have the potential to cause cancer. A high-fat diet also usually lacks dietary fiber, starch and plant foods that increase the "good" bacteria that keep cells in the colon healthy. A slow transit time with a low-fiber diet also means that carcinogens will spend a longer period of time in the colon.

Liver cancer can begin with high doses of alcohol that damages the liver cells.

Cancers of the breast, cervix, endometrium, and ovary have been linked with dietary fat and a high level of body fat in postmenopausal women, although not all studies find an association. High levels of body fat are accompanied by increased levels of estrogens. A high-fiber, low-fat diet, especially one with high quantities of vegetables rich in indoles, alters the chemistry of estrogens, making them less likely to increase the risk of cancer.

Polyunsaturated Fats

It's quite possible that fat may increase steroid hormones produced in the body or may exert its influence through prostaglandins. Fat may also cause cell membrane structures to become less resistant to carcinogens.

Epidemiological studies indicate strongly that certain types of fat play a role in cancers of the breast, colon, endometrium and prostate. Animal studies back some of these associations.

> **For example, polyunsaturated fatty acids promote carcinogenesis in animals more effectively than saturated fatty acids do, possibly because cancer cells use the essential fatty acid linoleic acid as fuel for their own growth. Such effects have not been noted in human populations, but this is not surprising, as they would be difficult to separate from confounding variables.**

For example, some of the polyunsaturated fat in our diets come from margarines that also contain compounds such as trans-fatty acids and hydrogenated fats, and these compounds are under suspicion as well.

In animals, diets with polyunsaturated fats are more closely associated with cancers in mammary glands and the pancreas, colon, skin, and liver than with saturated fats. We cannot apply these studies directly to humans, but they do give some warning signals.

> **It is most likely that specific fatty acids, or the balance of different kinds of fats, may create the greatest risk.**

For example, the ratio of omega 6 to omega 3 fatty acids may be relevant. An analysis in 1990 of the large-scale Multiple Risk Factor Intervention Trial conducted in the 1970s and 1980s showed a strong correlation between the ratio of these two types of polyunsaturated fats and cancer incidence and mortality. In practice, this means that a low intake of fish and vegetables combined with a high intake of polyunsaturated oils and margarines represents a potential hazard for the development of cancer. It is difficult, however, to put the blame wholly on any single food and there is no evidence that polyunsaturated fats themselves cause cancer. They may simply set up the right climate for cancers caused by something else to proliferate.

> **By the same token, olive oil, which is rich in monounsaturated fats, has been shown to provide protection against some cancers.**

Studies in Greece and Spain have found a lower incidence of breast cancer in women who consumed olive oil. Many of them used olive oil to make vegetables more appetizing, so it may have been their higher vegetable intake that protected them. It's important to note that some studies suggest that too much of any kind of fat may increase the risk of cancer in humans.

One widely publicized study maintained that fat was not related to breast cancer, since the incidence of breast cancer in women who had reduced their fat from 40 percent of calories from fat to 30 percent did not change. Other researchers have since pointed out that levels of fat may have to go much lower than this before dramatic differences are seen. Epidemiological comparisons of women in Western countries and in Asia suggest that those whose levels of fat fall below 25 percent of calories (a common percentage throughout Asia) are protected against breast cancer. However, these low levels of fat in the Asian diet are accompanied by a high intake of soy products and vegetables, and it may be these that are giving protection. Asian diets also tend to have low levels of meat.

Red Meat

Epidemiological studies show that those who eat a high-meat diet have higher levels of cancers of the breast, colon, pancreas, and prostate. However, it is difficult to separate the effects of meat fat from the meat itself. A high-meat diet may also have fewer vegetables and therefore fewer protective factors.

A well-conducted Harvard study reported that men who ate red meat as a main dish five or more times a week were 2.6 times as likely to suffer advanced prostate cancer as those who ate red meat once a week or less.

Other studies suggest it may be only processed meats that are likely to increase cancer risk. Against these theories, consider also that mammary tumors in rats, and stomach and skin cancers in mice, are reduced if the animals have a higher level of a fatty acid called conjugated linoleic acid (CLA), which occurs in cooked beef and lamb and in dairy products such as pasteurized milk, yogurt, and cheeses. CLA seems to have a role in preventing growth of cancers. It is possible that CLA may compete with and replace less desirable fats trying to get into cell membranes, or it may change messages within cells. Its role is still being explored—we do not yet have all the answers. The evidence condemning fat, and some foods that contain it, however, continues to grow. High levels of meat protein are under suspicion. Plant foods, by contrast, seem to offer protection against cancer.

Fat-reduced milk and yogurt may also provide some protection against bowel cancer, possibly because of their high content of calcium.

At this stage, the safest advice is to eat more vegetables and other plant foods and less fat, especially fewer omega 6 polyunsaturated fats, unless they are balanced with more of the omega 3 polyunsaturates found in fish and vegetables.

Antioxidants

The greatest body of cancer research is devoted to the study of fruits and vegetables and their potential to protect you against cancer. There are hundreds of studies showing that those who eat the most fruit and vegetables have the least cancer at almost every site in the body.

Smokers who eat the most fruit and vegetables are less likely to develop lung cancer compared with smokers who eat fewer fruits and vegetables, and most studies have also shown that cancers of the breast, colon, esophagus, stomach, pancreas, and various other sites have an inverse relationship with fruit and vegetable intake.

These foods are major sources of vitamin C and beta-carotene, and also have some vitamin E—all antioxidant substances. Some researchers jumped to the conclusion that these nutrients protect against cancer, but the results of an eight-year Finnish lung cancer trial in which 29,000 smokers were given supplements of these vitamins, either alone or in combination, casts doubt on this simplistic notion. This study—and another of 18,000 American smokers—showed that no benefit was gained by the supplements and that those taking beta-carotene had a significantly higher incidence of lung cancer than those given the placebo pills. Similar findings occurred from trials of beta-carotene and colonic polyps. It was a disappointment to those selling vitamin supplements, but these findings do not negate the original studies of fruit and vegetables—these foods may simply contain something else that provides protection.

Natural foods are amazingly complex mixtures of compounds, and a growing body of research is showing that many substances work quite differently when isolated from their companion compounds, as was shown in these studies of beta-carotene and cancer.

The original studies were not wrong in claiming protective effects from fruit and vegetables, but they wrongly assumed that the benefit came from vitamins. Fruit and vegetables contain several thousand different compounds.

Americans report eating 190 lbs. of fresh fruit and vegetables a year—much less than is required for adequate protection against cancer.

Here is a listing of just a few known antioxidants found in commonly available foods:

Antioxidant-Rich Foods

Food	Antioxidants present
Apples	bioflavonoids
Basil	O-cimene, cineol, esdragol
Broad beans	flavonoids (especially quercetin)
Broccoli	carotenoids, plant sterols, dithiolthiones, glucosinolates (indoles), isothiocyanates
Capers	biflavones, resins, glucosides
Capsicum	capsaicin, carotenoids
Carrots	carotenoids, coumarins, flavonoids
Citrus fruits	carotenoids, flavonoids, limonoids, coumarins, monoterpenes, triterpenoids
Eggplant	phenols, plant sterols, saponins
Fennel	phenols, esdragol, anethole
Garlic	glucosides, allyl methyl trisulphide, allylic sulphides, allicin, glutamyl, allylic cysteines
Ginger	curcumins, gingerols, diarylhptanoids
Horseradish	isothiocyanates
Flaxseeds	alpha-linolenic acid, lignans
Marjoram	terpineol, borneol, rosmarinic acid
Mint	menthol, cineol, menthoruran, terpenes
Olives and olive oil	phenols
Onions	flavonoids, many sulphur compounds
Oregano	thymol, terpenes, carnarole, ursolic acid
Parsley	coumarins, carotenoids (especially lutein), flavonoids, monoterpenes, phenols, phthalides, polyacetalenes,

98) *Good Fats, Bad Fats*

	apiin, pinene
Purslane	alpha-linolenic acid, carotenoids
Rosemary	pinene, borneol, carnosol, ursolic acid
Sage	borneol, camphor, cineol, tuyone, tannins, ursolic acid
Soybeans	phytestrogens, flavonoids
Tea	green or black, tannins, including polyphenols, catechins
Thyme	thymol, terpenes, tannins, carnarole
Tomatoes (red, ripe)	carotenoids, especially lycopene, coumarins (especially quercetin), plant sterols
Vegetables	carotenoids, numerous antioxidants
Wine, red	polyphenols, including resveratrol

Research is being done to isolate anticancer compounds in fruits and vegetables. It's a long task, as there are several thousand compounds to sift through and it is estimated that more than 600 may have anticancer activity. Other foods, including garlic, extra virgin olive oil, and chicken also contain anticancer compounds. Some compounds have been isolated. For example, broccoli contains sulforaphane, a dithiolthione compound that can block tumor formation in animals. Brussels sprouts, cauliflower, spring onions, and cabbage have it too, although in slightly smaller quantities.

It is unlikely that any single substance in fruits and vegetables is providing protection and it is unlikely that the protection will ever be available in a pill.

The chances are that many compounds may be involved and that synergistic effects between particular substances are important. At this stage, our only certainty is that eating *more* fruit and vegetables and *less* fat may offer some protection against most of the common cancers, especially colorectal cancer. This is almost certainly the diet to which humans are biologically adapted—not the highly processed fatty foods that make up so much of the diet for many people.

Lutein and Xeathanthin

Two carotenoids, lutein and xeathanthin, are also important in the macula of the eye, the region that permits us to see fine detail. Degeneration of the macula is the major cause of partial visual impairment and blindness that accompanies old age. Studies have already shown that those with low levels of these two carotenoids in their blood have a much greater risk of developing macular degeneration and blindness.

23

DIETARY FAT AND DIABETES

Diabetes is a serious, lifelong condition affecting about 16 million people in the United States.

Experts predict that by 2025, diabetes will strike 300 million adults worldwide.

Over a quarter of them aren't even aware they have it. Fortunately, many of the devastating complications that come with having this disease can be prevented in part by making sound nutritional changes.

Type 1, or insulin-dependent diabetes, occurs when the body doesn't make a hormone called insulin. It represents 5 to 10 percent of all cases. Insulin takes glucose out of your blood and carries it into your cells as a source of energy.

Type 2 Diabetes

The most common form of diabetes is type 2, or non-insulin-dependent diabetes mellitus (NIDDM). It is strongly related to dietary fat and approximately 90 percent of those with type 2 are overweight. If you have the gene for type 2 but stay slim, exercise regularly, and do not consume large quantities of certain fats, the disease will probably never appear. The majority of those who develop type 2 diabetes now have no known relative with the disease.

If a person becomes overweight, the fat in cells produces a hormone called "resistin," which interferes with the action of insulin so that the condition called insulin resistance develops. Insulin is then unable to do its job. The pancreas tries to compensate by producing more insulin, but gradually the overworked gland will malfunction and its ability to secrete insulin may falter. As type 2 develops, the production of insulin declines.

> One of the consequences of having diabetes and being overweight is that the need for insulin is compounded. Excess body fat requires more insulin to maintain normal levels of glucose.

Because glucose isn't able to get into the fat cells, it builds up in the blood, eventually spilling over into the urine as the body excretes it. It truly is a vicious cycle: increased body fat can lead to insulin resistance and type 2 diabetes, which in turn may increase the appetite and lead to overeating. Exercise helps in the treatment of type 2 diabetes, as it helps break down the barriers of fat around the cells. Weight loss also helps, and the easiest way to accomplish this is to cut back on calories, especially those from sugar, fat, and alcohol.

Monounsaturated Fats

Some studies show that diabetes improves if the diet includes a moderate level of fat, mainly monounsaturated fat from a product such as olive oil, plus ample quantities of fish. Most people with diabetes found such a diet easier to stick to than one that had very low levels of fat and more carbohydrate.

After a meal, the fats you consume show up in your blood as triglycerides. Some hours later, the triglycerides should have been cleared from your blood and either used for energy or tucked away in fat stores. In type 2, high levels of triglycerides are usually still circulating in the blood after an overnight fast.

The treatment for high triglyceride levels is to cut back on saturated fats and reduce the consumption of alcohol and refined sugar. Many researchers also believe it is best to avoid high levels of polyunsaturated fats, and to switch to monounsaturated fats.

24

DIETARY FAT AND GALLSTONES

Gallstones are common in our country and one in ten Americans develop them. Some of us are genetically predisposed to developing them. They are more common in women between the ages twenty and sixty, who are twice as likely to develop them as men.

> **Among the Pima Indians of Arizona, there is a genetic tendency to produce bile with large amounts of cholesterol, and 70 percent of women have gallstones by the time they reach the age of 30.**

Overweight and obese women are especially at risk. Researchers have found that being just moderately overweight increases the risk of gallstones. That may be because excess body fat can reduce the amount of bile salts in the gallbladder that causes more cholesterol production. The rate also increases with people who eat a lot of fat, including (some claim *especially*) polyunsaturated fats.

Your gallbladder is situated behind the lower ribs on the right side of your body. It stores bile, a golden-brown fluid produced by your liver for digesting fats. After a meal, your gallbladder squirts bile into your small intestine.

Gallstones can form when high levels of cholesterol in bile precipitate and combine with calcium salts to form stones. One or many stones may form, and they can vary from the size of a grain of sand to the size of a golf ball, or even larger.

Many people have "silent stones," or gallstones that don't cause symptoms and never develop any. Others have a sudden, severe, steady pain in the upper abdomen, chest, between the shoulders or pain under the right shoulder and may be accompanied by nausea and vomiting. These symptoms may last for minutes or several hours. In some cases, the pain is mild and feels more like indigestion. If a stone blocks the duct that joins the gallbladder to the main bile duct, the gallbladder can become inflamed, causing fever and severe pain on the right side of the abdomen. This is called cholecystitis.

As gallstones are made in the gallbladder, its removal, along with the stones, will resolve the symptoms and prevent any more stones from developing. You have the ability to live well without a gallbladder. Bile simply passes from the liver directly to the intestine instead of being stored in the gallbladder.

Some studies suggest that removal of the gallbladder can cause high blood cholesterol, so it's a good idea to check your cholesterol levels occasionally if you have had yours removed. Conversely, cholesterol-lowering drugs can actually increase the amount of cholesterol in bile and so increase risk of gallstones in some people.

A low-fat, high-fiber diet reduces the risk of getting gallstones in the first place. If you have them already, diet or nutritional supplements cannot dissolve them. Many times a gallstone attack occurs after a fatty meal; however, the pain is related to the attack rather than to specific foods. There is no need to avoid eggs or anything else except high-fat foods. It makes sense, however, not to overdo fatty foods of any kind. Fast weight loss and fasting can increase the risk of gallstones.

PART IV

Fat-Free Fats

Almost everyone now knows that fats are fattening. Some are also aware that certain fats can contribute to heart disease, high blood pressure, diabetes, gallstones, and some cancers. Yet most people throughout the world are consuming more and more foods high in fat. For some, high-fat foods are such an intrinsic part of their diet that they cannot consider going without them. You may be looking for foods that look and taste as though they are rich in fat but have little or none of the genuine article.

25

ARE FAKE FATS
MAKING US FATTER?

A survey conducted by the Calorie Control Council found that two-thirds of us feel there is a need for fat replacements. The food industry has spent millions of dollars and years of research trying to come up with fat-free fat to fill that demand. They want something that looks like fat, rolls around in the mouth like fat, slips down the throat creamily as fat does—but does not have the calories that normal fats provide.

The market for fat replacers and fake fats is growing rapidly.

> Eighty-seven percent of all adults eat either reduced-fat or low-fat, sugar-free products. Grocery store shelves are bulging under the sheer volume of "light" products, and this market will only continue to expand.

Despite the plethora of these products, however, Americans of all ages and both sexes continue to grow fatter.

With an increasing percentage of the population becoming overweight, however, and more people feeling paranoid about all fat, there is a strong chance that more such products could become common throughout the developed world.

> One in four Americans are on diets, while another third say they are making significant efforts to control their weight.

The food industry knows that we want to have our cake and eat it too. It's in their best interest to try to meet our demands. Manufacturers look for soluble, colorless, and flavorless fat substitutes carrying various properties that are all compatible with other ingredients in the product. For example, if some of the fat is removed from a food such as margarine, it will be replaced by water, and a fat substitute will have to keep the water combined with the remaining fat so that the product retains its texture and spreadability. Some efforts at fat-reduced margarines failed because the products melted too readily and their increased water content made foods such as hot toast go soggy.

No single fat substitute works for all products. Low-fat whipped yogurt and soft ice cream usually use a gum, rather than water, to hold air in the product. Other foods such as some types of confectionery need a poly-alcohol product that will resist the crystallization of sugars in the product. For many fat-reduced foods, a combination of fat substitutes is usually necessary to achieve all the characteristics desired such as creaminess, mouth feel, processing stability, the ability to hold air and water, and bulk.

26

OLESTRA

Not long ago, a top chef in the United States prepared a meal of thick seafood soup, herb-crusted fried duck breast, fried trout, fried softshell crayfish, salad with vinaigrette dressing, and a rich cake. Each dish was prepared with lots of oil. Such a meal would usually contain more than 100 grams of fat. In this meal, however, each dish was prepared with olestra, an oil made from a fake fat that was approved by the Food and Drug Administration in 1996. The fat content of this experimental olestra-rich meal was minimal.

> **Procter & Gamble first submitted olestra to the FDA for approval in 1975 as a cholesterol-lowering drug. However, it fell short of meeting the necessary criteria.**

In the United States, olestra is approved for use in a range of snack foods, including potato chips, tortilla chips, and crackers. The manufacturer is pursuing approval in Canada and the United Kingdom. Olestra is not yet used in Europe, and many nutritionists and consumer advocates hope it won't be given a green light because it could be one of the biggest disasters ever to hit our food supply.

The Whole Ball of Wax

Olestra is marketed under the brand name Olean. Technically, it is known as a sucrose polyester, sometimes written as SPE, and just like any polyester it is a molecule manufactured in a laboratory. It does not occur naturally. Fats are usually made up of triglycerides—three fatty acid molecules attached to a form of alcohol known as glycerol, as described in Chapter 2. Olestra was developed when scientists began tinkering with the number of fatty acids and discovered that an increase in fatty acids decreased the body's ability to digest and absorb the fat.

> **By replacing glycerol with sucrose that is protected by six, seven, or eight fatty acid bodyguards, fat-splitting enzymes can't get to the sucrose center in order to break it down.**

Unlike some other substitute products, olestra has a wide range of uses that are very similar to fat. Although it has been approved as a fat replacement only in salty snack foods, its chemical makeup would withstand frying, spreading on toast, or as an ingredient in baked goods, pizzas, fast foods, candy, ice cream, sauces, mayonnaise, and margarine. It has no flavor of its own, but in foods it attracts flavors in much the same way other fats do. In the mouth, it tastes like an oil.

The texture, taste, and mouth feel are remarkably like many other processed tasteless fats, although those with a sensitive palate can detect foods that are cooked in olestra. The newspaper *USA Today* asked forty-four people who happened to be passing by to taste potato chips cooked either in olestra or in the usual fat. They were not told which was which, but twenty-five people correctly identified the chips cooked in olestra. Many thought the difference was slight, and few objected. While this did not involve enough people to make it scientifically valid, it is always interesting to see spontaneous tests done by ordinary people and not by someone trying to market a product.

Digestive Woes

Because olestra is not recognized by human digestive enzymes, it passes through the body without contributing any calories or cholesterol. That sounds ideal, but olestra's passage through the gastrointestinal tract can cause problems.

> **Some of these, such as bloating, abdominal pain, and loose stools, may appear within hours of eating it, while for others it may take 20 to 30 years to become apparent. It is these potential long-term effects that worry many nutritionists.**

In some people, olestra passes to the large bowel to be excreted along with other waste products. In others, it may simply ooze through the digestive system and be discharged when you least expect it. The company making olestra has spent a lot of time and money, and has changed the viscosity of the product to reduce the likelihood of this problem. The product in its oil form now looks rather like Vaseline. In spite of the changes, however, the Food and Drug Administration still requires products containing olestra to carry a warning that "olestra may cause abdominal cramping and loose stools."

Olestra's manufacturers claim that only a small percentage of people suffer undesirable gastrointestinal effects, but this is disputed by some researchers who believe that this percentage is larger. The quantity consumed will obviously have some influence on the potential problem, and if such fake fats are added to a wide variety of foods, or used in excessive quantities as described in the meal at the beginning of this chapter, a much higher percentage of people are likely to suffer abdominal cramping and loose stools.

> **In test studies where people were given 32 grams of olestra a day in muffins, dinner rolls, and other foods, almost one-quarter developed diarrhea.**

Other informal surveys gave people a small serving of potato chips that contained either regular fat or olestra, without the recipients knowing which type they were getting. None of those who had regular chips had gastrointestinal changes, whereas one-sixth of those whose potato chips contained olestra had bloating or loose stools.

Chipping Away at Our Nutrients

It is of some consolation that the abdominal effects will at least stop most people who experience them from consuming any more products containing olestra. More serious is the fact that on its way through the gastrointestinal tract, olestra may also take with it the fat-soluble vitamins A, D, E, and K. The manufacturers of olestra, to their credit, have been concerned about this and are adding these vitamins to snack foods that contain olestra.

> The FDA requires a label statement on foods telling consumers that "olestra inhibits the absorption of some vitamins and other nutrients. Vitamins A, D, E, and K have been added."

The major problem is that vitamins A and D are potentially dangerous in excess. If olestra is added to a broader range of foods, how can we control the total dose?

Vitamin A

Too much vitamin A is hazardous in pregnancy and has been shown to increase the risk of deformities in the fetus. It is difficult to take in too much of these vitamins from natural sources because they are found in a rather limited number of foods, and usually not in large quantities. The richest source of vitamin A is liver, and some medical authorities think pregnant women should avoid it just in case some eat an excessive quantity. The chances of overconsuming snack foods containing olestra and added vitamin A would be much greater.

> **All products with olestra and added vitamin A should therefore carry a warning that they must not be consumed by pregnant women. Young children might also need some restriction of their vitamin A intake.**

Vitamin D

Vitamin D normally comes from the action of sunlight on a substance in skin. Tanning of the skin exerts a natural control over excess vitamin D being made in this way because it slows the reaction. Adding vitamin D to foods, however, is potentially hazardous. Just five to ten times the recommended daily allowance (RDA) is dangerous. Olestra can cause substantial losses of vitamin D from the body, but if the fake fat were used in many foods, and each had extra vitamin D to make up for the losses olestra causes, it would be virtually impossible to control the intake of vitamin D.

> **Even if the product's label recommended limits on how much of it consumers of different ages and sizes should eat, the total vitamin D intake would depend on how many foods containing olestra were consumed each day.**

In practice, adding vitamin D to a range of foods is not feasible. For this reason alone, some people consider olestra a hazard in the food supply.

Carotenoids

Potentially, there is an even more serious problem. Olestra can also remove from the body some of the protective carotenoid substances occurring in fruits and vegetables. There is strong evidence that these substances function as anticancer agents, protecting DNA from the damage that increases the risks of many types of cancer.

Hundreds of studies have shown that those who eat the most fruits and vegetables have the lowest incidence of cancer at almost every site in the body. Over fifty studies have specifically shown that diets rich in the wide variety of carotenoids found in fruits and vegetables are associated with a lower risk of cancers.

Researchers in the Netherlands reported that small quantities of olestra significantly depleted carotenoids.

They included modest quantities of olestra in a margarine and measured the effect on five different carotenoids and vitamin E levels in the body. Their report stated that "even at low doses, sucrose polyester strongly reduces plasma carotenoid concentrations."

Many of the carotenoids need some fat for their absorption. For example, lycopene, which occurs in tomatoes and watermelons and protects against prostate cancer, is absorbed better from a meal that also contains some fat. Using a fake fat such as olestra may interfere directly with the absorption of lycopene, and also reduce absorption because it has been substituted for a real fat.

You may not need much olestra to wipe out the value of these natural protective agents.

Currently, the FDA is reviewing studies that look at how olestra is affecting the absorption of carotenoids. Olestra's supporters don't feel there is enough proof that carotenoids are valuable natural anticancer substances. It would take decades of research to prove they are wrong, and we cannot gamble with people's lives and health in this way.

Beta Carotene

The best-known carotenoid is beta-carotene, often called pro-vitamin A, which the body converts to vitamin A. Until recently, other carotenoids were largely ignored because they do not form vitamin A and were therefore thought to have no benefit for humans. Researchers have since found that these other carotenoids in fruits and vegetables protect against some cancers, whereas betacarotene may not do so.

Two major trials, in which beta-carotene was given as a supplement, found an *increase* in the incidence of lung cancer, and two other trials have found an increase in bowel polyps, the precursors to bowel cancer. There is some evidence that a carotenoid called lycopene may give protection against cancer, but even this is an educated guess, not proof. Researchers don't yet know conclusively which of the carotenoids in fruits and vegetables give the best protection. Your body may need all, or at least many of them, and singling out just one is no guarantee of safety. Health authorities therefore unanimously recommend that we increase our consumption of a variety of fruits and vegetables.

The anticancer compounds in fruits and vegetables don't make us immune to cancer but they help the body's immune system fight cancer-causing substances that come from cigarette smoking, pollution, and, possibly, too much of some kinds of fat. They also protect against coronary heart disease and cataracts, and other eye problems associated with aging.

We simply don't know what the long-term effects of olestra are. We do know that, so far, it has reduced the body's levels of every carotenoid tested. As there are more than 600 of these substances, complete test results are almost impossible. As consumers, we must all question whether a food company should have the right to add something to foods that may turn out to have such profoundly dreadful effects on health, especially when the substance is being added only so we can stuff ourselves with more food than our bodies need.

Unlike other food additives, olestra is not taken into the body in milligram or microgram doses but in grams—

hundreds or even thousands of times the dose of most food additives. Every substance known is toxic if the dose is large enough.

Are We Slimmer Yet?

If olestra is allowed to be used in a wide range of products, most would be marketed as guilt-free binge foods. Eating foods that are fat-free can dissolve the usual restraint we have around high-fat foods, and cause us to eat too freely. It's easy to consume large amounts of products that taste fatty and provide fewer calories.

If you find it difficult to reign in your appetite for snacks, it would be wise to avoid olestra altogether.

Lots of us love guilt-free fat now, but what if research finds a link between fake fats and cancer or cataracts in twenty or thirty years? We would be justified in blaming those who allowed such products to be sold in the first place, especially when doubts are already being publicized by concerned individuals and consumer groups.

Many dieters enjoy being able to tuck into fat-free potato chips containing olestra, but in doing so they are ignoring warnings from groups such as the Center for Science in the Public Interest (CSPI), a consumer health advocacy group, and the American Public Health Association. CSPI maintains that we don't have enough evidence that olestra won't be harmful in the long term. Health authorities should be required to give those facts more weight than the potential profits for food manufacturers who want to be able to use olestra in their products.

27

OTHER FAKE FATS

Olestra has created great interest and consternation among many nutritionists and consumer groups, but it is not the only fake fat. In fact, the first fat substitute, Avicel, was approved in the mid-1960s. Since then, others have followed and are now commonly used by manufacturers. Several more are in the pipeline. The older types are carbohydrate products based on starch derivatives or gums that can hold water—these types are used when some of the fat in a product is replaced by water. Others are substitutes for fat, and some newer ones are fats that have been manipulated by food technologists so that they cannot be absorbed by the body.

Carbohydrate-Based Fat Substitutes

Sorbitol, xylitol, mannitol, isomalt, polydextrose, and maltodextrins have been used for some years to replace fats in some processed foods. They are useful for maintaining the structure of some products and for providing bulk, texture, and mouth feel when fat is removed.

Sugar alcohols have some sweetness as well as an ability to absorb water and act as fat substitutes in certain foods, so they are often used. Unlike the sugars from which they are derived, these compounds do not contribute to dental decay.

Sorbitol

This is the oldest of the sugar alcohols, first made in 1872 from the mountain ash berry. Sorbitol also occurs naturally in cherries, plums, seaweed, apples, and pears, but when it is used as a food additive for pastries, cakes, and candy, it is made in the laboratory by the hydrogenation of glucose, sucrose, or starch. It contributes 2.6 calories per gram, and it breaks down more slowly in the body than sugar does. It has less than a third of the calories in a gram of fat. Products containing sorbitol and other sugar alcohols can cause diarrhea if consumed in large quantities. The labels of products containing these ingredients warn that excess consumption can have a laxative effect. The high content of sorbitol in natural apple juice is a major cause of diarrhea in young children who consume apple juice as their major liquid.

Xylitol

This is another naturally occurring sugar alcohol that acts as a bulking agent in some fat-reduced foods. Although it can be extracted from raspberries, strawberries, some types of plums, lettuce, mushrooms, cauliflower, and seaweed, xylitol is now processed from wood pulp (especially from birch trees); from the shells of almonds, coconuts, or pecans; from the hulls of oats, rice, or cottonseed; or from sugar cane refuse. The extraction process forms a sugar compound called xylose, then is hydrogenated, purified and crystallized to form a white powder. Xylitol is added to foods such as chewing gum and candy and has 2.4 calories per gram. It is perhaps the sweetest of all sugar alcohols. Like sorbitol, too much can cause diarrhea.

Mannitol

Often used in chewing gum, mannitol, or manna sugar as it is sometimes called, can be produced from seaweed, the wood pulp of coniferous trees, the dried exudate of the manna tree, or from various sugars. It also causes diarrhea in large doses and makes some children nauseated. Each gram contains 1.6 calories.

Isomalt

This sugar alcohol is made from ordinary sugar, or sucrose. It is a white, sweet-tasting crystalline powder that supposedly intensifies other flavors without having any flavor of its own. It acts as a substitute for sugar and fat in foods. Manufacturers commonly use it to sweeten beverages, candy, chewing gum, and jellies and jams. It has 2 calories per gram.

Polydextrose

Formed by combining glucose, sorbitol, and a small amount of citric acid, polydextrose is a carbohydrate polymer that does not taste sweet. Each gram contributes 1 calorie. Polydextrose is used in chewing gum, salad dressings, gelatins, fat-reduced yogurt, ice cream, baked goods, and to replace some of the fat in fat-reduced chocolate. One brand of polydextrose already appearing in foods is branded as Litesse.

Maltodextrins

These are made from various starches derived from corn, potato, rice, tapioca, or a mixture of several grains, and there are dozens of different maltodextrin compounds available. In foods, they can act like a cross between sugar and starch and contribute 4 calories per gram. Many maltodextrins are used in cakes, breads, desserts, ice cream, fat-reduced spreads, cheese products, dips, mayonnaise, dressings, and candy. Some types are good at binding fats, adding a creamy texture that becomes slimy if too little is used. One product commonly used is called CrystaLean.

Emulsifiers and Gums

Some or all of the fat in some foods can be replaced by emulsifiers and gums (lecithin, guar, locust bean, tragacanth, acacia, karaya) that keep water and fat evenly dispersed throughout products such as margarine, peanut butter, salad dressings, and mayonnaise. They are also used to increase the quantity of air trapped in some foods such as ice cream, or to keep products such as cakes and breads soft. Emulsifiers may be vegetable gums, compounds derived from sorbitol, or mono- and diglycerides made from vegetable oils. Some of the emulsifiers and gums used by the food industry may sound familiar:

Lecithin

This phospholipid is produced in the body as well as occurring naturally in foods such as soybeans and egg yolks. It is commonly used as an emulsifier to bind ingredients that don't normally mix in candy bars, mayonnaise, sauces, drinks, soups, peanut butter, spreads, and desserts.

Guar

This plant produces a gummy fibrous substance that expands when it comes into contact with moisture. At one time the gum was promoted in weight-loss supplements but has since been found to be a choking hazard. Food manufacturers use guar gum to thicken and stabilize foods such as sauces and ice cream.

Locust Bean

The gum from this plant is also called carob gum or St. John's bread. It binds water and increases the elasticity of some products. It is used in processed cheese, bakery products, and ice cream.

Tragacanth

This bush, from the genus Astragalus, produces a gum that swells in water and forms a paste. It is used as a suspending agent in no-oil salad dressings, fruit fillings, and citrus beverages.

Acacia

Gum arabic is exuded by wounds in the bark of Acacia trees. It prevents fats forming a greasy film in foods and is also used as a cloud agent in beverages.

Karaya

The Sterculia urens tree, a native of India, produces a gum that swells in water. It is used to give body to low-fat toppings, frozen desserts, and baked goods. It is also used as a denture adhesive!

Protein-Based Fat Substitutes

Lita

This reduced-calorie product is made from protein. This time a protein called zein, found in corn, is the raw material. Its structure resembles fat, but it contributes only 1 calorie per gram.

Caprenin

This fat substitute has some of the characteristics of chocolate but carries just 5 calories per gram. It is commonly used as a substitute for cocoa butter in candy bars. It is made by combining glycerol with three fatty acids, one of which cannot be properly absorbed by the body, so its use is limited. Health authorities are having some difficulties with caprenin. Because it is made from fatty acids that occur elsewhere in nature, its manufacturers claim that it does not need special clearance as a food additive. However, caprenin's three particular fatty acids do not occur together in nature, so it may have some characteristics not yet understood.

Whenever some food additive is not absorbed, it must pass through the gastrointestinal tract. In doing so, it may either have some effect on other foods or nutrients or it may alter some types of normal, and beneficial, bacteria.

Simplesse

A chance discovery some years ago found that fat substitutes can also be made from protein. When tiny protein particles are sheared off from whey protein (a byproduct in cheese-making) during simultaneous pasteurization and homogenization, they form small uniform round particles. In the mouth, these tiny spherical balls formed from milk or egg protein roll around, and their mouth feel resembles that of fat. The process is called microparticulation and the particles are so small that 50 billion could fit onto a teaspoon. Their small size gives a feeling of creaminess in the mouth. Larger particles would feel powdery or gritty. The process has been patented and a product made largely by mixing egg white and skim milk has been registered with the name Simplesse. You may know it more intimately as the fat substitute in some frozen desserts. A 4-ounce serving may contain as little as 1 gram of fat, whereas the same amount of regular ice cream has 13 grams. Since only small quantities of Simplesse are used, its energy contribution is low.

Simplesse is also used to replace the fat in sour cream, yogurt, mayonnaise, dips, and spreads; some cheese substitutes for products such as pizza have also been developed.

Some other forms of Simplesse have been developed for bakery products, soups, and products that must be heated, but the major problem for Simplesse is that it breaks down with heat so it can't be used for frying.

32

Do We Need Fat Substitutes?

According to some experts, almost two-thirds of us think that we do. Makers of fake fats claim that their products are useful for reducing calories and fat in the daily diet. Some cite the fact that saturated fats contribute to high blood cholesterol and assume that products with fat substitutes will help to lower cholesterol levels in the body. There is no proof of this. There is no proof that fake fats help you to lose weight and there is some evidence that they do not. As these products have proliferated in our country, the population has grown steadily fatter.

Some spokespeople for the manufacturers of fake fats claim that increasing obesity is due to decreasing levels of physical activity. There is no doubt that this is correct if we look back over the last ten, twenty, or thirty years. Levels of activity have not fallen, however, over the last few years since fat and sugar substitutes have been available, but our population has grown steadily fatter.

There are several possible reasons for the rise in obesity: perhaps overweight people do not use fat-modified products; or perhaps using foods with fake fats induces guilt-free comfort about consuming a greater overall quantity of food.

> **Some studies support this and show that total calorie intake does not decrease when people consume fat and sugar substitutes.**

Foods containing fake fats are not free of calories. They may have fewer calories, but a 2-ounce serving of olestra-fried potato chips still has 150 calories. The calorie count is half the level in regular chips but is still significant, especially if you eat twice as many chips! In such cases, there would be virtually no saving in calories and a large load of olestra to pass through the intestine. If you ate other foods also containing olestra, your total daily intake could be very high.

The problem of people compensating for fake ingredients by eating larger quantities of foods is well documented. People simply eat more to make up for what they have omitted.

> **Sugar substitutes have been well studied and there is plenty of evidence that people using them unconsciously eat more of other foods.**

We are eating four times the amount of sugar substitutes as we were over twenty years ago, but our sugar consumption has gone up as well. Obviously sugar substitutes haven't decreased our use of sugar. Will fat substitutes fare better?

While there are no proven benefits and even a small shadow of doubt hanging over some fake fats, it is difficult to justify their use. To add to their difficulties, fat substitutes cannot duplicate all the characteristics of fats. For example, a genuine ice cream needs not only the texture and mouth feel of cream but also its complex flavor. Even combinations of several substitutes cannot hope to match the unique richness of dairy fats. Similarly, the flavor of a good olive oil is integral to a mayonnaise or salad dressing, and no fat-free substitute can duplicate such complexity of flavor. One of the most difficult foods for technologists to produce in fat-reduced form is cheese. It can be done to a certain extent in processed cheeses, but many true cheese lovers do not eat these products. Cheese connoisseurs doubt that anyone could ever replace the unique flavors and mouth feel of a good cheese. They also ask why anyone would want to. We could all ask the same question.

> Do we seek fat substitutes so that we can continue to
> stuff ourselves with vast quantities of food without get-
> ting fat? It isn't possible to eat vast quantities of food
> with fat substitutes without gaining weight.

The development of fake fats has helped perpetuate the myth
that fat is inherently bad. Some fats are. It is probably fair to say
that for many adults, saturated fats have little to recommend
them, although they can supply a very palatable form of energy
for those who *need* more calories. Red meat and dairy products,
which are high in saturated fat, are also excellent sources of iron
and calcium, nutrients that are often missing from our diets
today. But all fats are not bad. Seeds, nuts, avocado, fatty fish,
and olive oil contain valuable and essential fats that could never
be replaced with fake substitutes, nor should they be.

Junk Knowledge

Many of the foods that contain problem fats are junk foods.
Replacing their fat does not give them nutritional credibility.
And there is always the possibility that food additives that are
totally foreign to the human gastrointestinal tract may prove to
be undesirable in twenty years' time. Even if the fake fats turn
out to be safe, the foods containing them are still products that
take the place of other more nutritious foods. If you eat junk
foods only as occasional extras, they won't cause any problems
and their fats do not need to be replaced.

Food authorities are concerned mainly with the safety of
food additives and ingredients. They do not consider such
questions as whether the product is necessary, makes sense, or
contributes any health benefit to the nation. With olestra,
many eminent scientists consider that even the safety issues are
unclear. For the longest study of olestra—taking thirty-nine
weeks—the subjects were pigs. Food technologists are trying to

gain an intimate understanding of the way different fat substitutes can be combined to provide textures, mouth feel, and the processing characteristics they desire—with fewer calories than fats provide. An alternative would be to abandon such pursuits and persuade people to eat the real thing but in smaller quantities. This obviously does not suit marketing people from companies who want to produce an ever-expanding range of profitable products. It might, however, be a more justifiable use of resources.

PART V

Dietary Fat and Body Fat

Humans need body fat. It pads our joints, and cushions organs such as the kidneys. Body fat also acts as a reserve of fuel to provide energy in times of scarce food supply or illness. Some body fat is also considered aesthetically pleasing, especially in women, possibly because it is a sign of fertility.

29

WALKING A THIN LINE

Desirable levels of body fat are influenced by fashion. In modern Western society, most women wish they were thinner. Indoctrinated by media images that a desirable body is lean, many young women go to extreme lengths to minimize their body fat. Many are constantly miserable because they cannot achieve the thinness they consider desirable. Concerns that body fat is ugly have now extended to the absurdity of many normal-weight girls as young as nine or ten developing an intense fear of fat. Athletes and their coaches also want the body pared down to its lean muscle, with as little extra weight to carry as possible. This preoccupation with body weight has increased the incidence of eating disorders.

Anorexia nervosa has existed for centuries, although it was once rare. Over the last thirty years or so, the incidence has increased and some studies show up to 1 percent of teenage girls are affected.

Some male athletes strive to reduce fat levels to 4 to 8 percent of their body weight. A few runners aim for body fat levels as low as 3 percent to reduce the load they carry while running, and to get rid of insulation so they can dissipate heat more easily. The equivalent level for female athletes would be 12 percent body fat. Exercise physiologists warn that such low levels of body fat, in men or women, pose the danger of a reduced capacity for exercise and greater likelihood of injury and illness.

Most women stop menstruating when body fat levels fall. At

least 16 percent fat is needed for menstruation to occur at all, and approximately 22 percent body fat is usually needed for a regular menstrual cycle. At lower levels of body fat, ovulation may occur only occasionally, so those female athletes who do not menstruate but don't want to become pregnant must take contraceptive precautions.

Bone Loss

While lack of fertility may not concern an actively competing female athlete, the low levels of estrogen that accompany it result in a loss of calcium from bone. These losses usually occur at menopause, when estrogen supplies normally fall and the risk of osteoporosis increases dramatically. Five to seven years after menstruation ceases, women will lose up to 20 percent of their bone mass. The longer women live, the greater their bone loss and the higher their chance of a serious fracture. There are over 1.5 million osteoporosis-related fractures every year. Most occur in women, but elderly men are also affected. The best prevention is to build a strong skeleton early in life, when more calcium can be absorbed into bone, and then maintain this with a good level of calcium and physical activity.

The process of bone loss begins at whatever age women are when they stop menstruating.

> **Studies on bone density of female athletes show alarming levels of osteoporosis even while they are in their late teen years and early twenties.**

No amount of exercise or calcium intake can protect them against such high calcium losses while their hormone levels are low.

Young women need to build dense bones to withstand the inevitable losses associated with aging after menopause. Very thin young women, whether athletes or not, have a double problem. Not only do they begin to lose bone density many years earlier than other women do, they miss the opportune time during their younger years to build up bone density. One of the best preventive measures you can take against osteoporosis is to keep body-fat levels at least normal, or slightly above normal, to maintain hormone levels. If you keep body fat at a healthy level and couple that with an adequate calcium intake and some weight-bearing exercise, you are employing the best defense against osteoporosis.

It is ironic that many young women diet to reduce body fat to look more attractive, yet the loss of bone density that accompanies their slenderness will cause a stooped, painful posture within ten to twenty years. A young woman of seventeen who reduces her body-fat level enough for her periods to cease may think she looks attractive now, but she can expect to spend much of her life looking *less* attractive than those carrying more fat but possessing a straight, strong spine.

Beyond Measure

Although percentage of body fat has begun to dominate the thinking of many men and women in our country, it is very hard to measure it accurately. Some health care professionals and fitness trainers use calipers to estimate skinfold thickness at various body sites and then use a formula to calculate body fat. Skinfold measurements are notoriously difficult to take accurately, and the formula has been discredited for its inaccuracy. This has not stopped people quoting body-fat levels determined by these methods. Underwater weighing can measure body fat more accurately, but the equipment is expensive and bulky, so this technique isn't commonly available to most people. It seems more sensible to stop quoting body-fat percentages. If fitness centers would help by no longer using such flawed measurements and formulas, many people may be less likely to dwell on exact body-fat percentage and think more about keeping the body in basic good shape.

30

TOO MUCH BODY FAT

It is undesirable to be too thin, but it is also hazardous to be too fat, especially if the excess fat is around your waist and on your upper body. A certain level of body fat is essential for the adequate production of female hormones, but there does not seem to be a similar role for extra fat on men. Excess fat on males is commonly deposited in fat stores in the abdomen, known as visceral fat. There is a strong body of evidence that this fat is a health hazard, increasing the risk of coronary heart disease, high blood pressure, diabetes, and some types of cancer. Health surveys show that almost 107 million American adults are too fat, with almost 44 million rated as obese.

Men

Overweight men were rare in most societies until recent times, when the food supply had become assured and physical effort was no longer necessary to collect food. Since machinery has been used for most physically demanding tasks, and most men drive cars instead of walking or cycling, the number with excess visceral fat has increased dramatically. An alarming 61 percent of American men, from age twenty to seventy-four, are considered overweight or obese. And, as men age, they tend to gain more weight around the abdomen than both pre- and post-menopausal women. Among men over age eighteen, 21 percent do not engage in any leisure-time physical activity and by age seventy-five, a third of American men have no leisure time physical activity at all.

Women

Overweight and obese women aged twenty to seventy-four and older make up 51 percent of our population. As with men, women are also prone to weight gain as they get older. Most women have fat around their hips and thighs during their reproductive years, which usually don't present a health risk. In fact, women at this state of life who are overweight but don't carry their weight around the abdomen are less likely to have health problems. During their forties and fifties, however, women tend to collect body fat. Many women think this has something to do with changing hormone levels, but it is more likely because they are less physically active once their children have grown up. Caring for children and the extra household tasks they create uses up energy, so that when these physical demands are no longer required, women tend to gain body fat. When children leave home, many women also eat out more. Few older women exercise regularly, so their total energy expenditure goes down while their input increases.

> Among women over 18 years of age, 27 percent have no leisure time activity, and this increases with age so that by the age of 75, one in two women do not do any exercise.

Body fat begins to accumulate slowly some years before menopause, but it is not until 8 or 10 pounds have settled that most women realize this weight gain has become a permanent part of their body. This realization usually coincides with menopause. However, diminishing hormones shouldn't be a scapegoat for those unwanted menopausal pounds. Women gain much the same amount of weight whether or not they use hormone replacement therapy—more evidence that the weight gain has more to do with aging and reduced physical activity than with changing hormone levels.

In affluent countries, high levels of body fat in both sexes and all ages are due to a lack of exercise and a modern food supply that is high in fat. Eating fat is the main cause of fat being deposited in the first place, although once excess fat is in place, calories from any source will prevent its loss.

> Studies show that most people underestimate their food intake, and overweight people underestimate more than those of normal weight do. Since fat hit the headlines as being undesirable, most people are even less likely to report their true intake, so that finding out how much fat people really eat is now difficult.

31

WHAT MAKES US FAT?

Nutritionists once believed that too many calories from any source would add to body fat. We now know that this is not true. Proteins are not stored and are rarely converted to fat and the body is not able to convert alcohol to fat.

Carbohydrates

Until recently, carbohydrates have borne the brunt of the blame for excess body fat, but research from several laboratories now confirms their innocence. It takes more energy for the body to convert carbohydrates to fat than it does to convert fat to fat. Your body prefers the more efficient process of turning dietary fat to body fat. When your body maintains a stable weight, it does not store much carbohydrate apart from some stored in muscles as glycogen and a smaller quantity as liver glycogen. Some carbohydrate goes to replenish blood glucose levels and the rest stimulates the body to burn more energy.

> Humans don't convert carbohydrate to fat until the daily intake exceeds 500 grams—the amount in 40 slices of bread, 11 cups of cooked rice, or 9 baked potatoes!

In practice, you do not usually get fat from eating carbohydrate-rich foods, *unless* those foods have added fat, which can be converted to body fat. This is different from the situation in other animals, where carbohydrates are readily converted to fat. But then, few animals eat a diet high in fat. Even carnivorous animals, which eat only animal flesh, will not get much fat if the animals they are eating are wild.

By contrast, many of the foods we eat—including many carbohydrate-rich foods—are high in fat. Bread, rice, potatoes, and pasta have little fat, but we put butter or margarine on the bread, fry the rice, add sour cream or butter to potatoes, or fry them in fat, and smother pasta in either creamy sauces or add loads of fatty meat and cheese. We then blame the bread, rice, potatoes, or pasta for making us fat.

> **It is not necessary to restrict carbohydrate foods unless they are also high in fat.**

The only exception to this would be sweetened drinks and candy. Neither contributes important nutrients, and while the body is burning their calories, it won't burn calories from fat. With the exception of sugar, most foods high in carbohydrate are also bulky, and this effectively restricts consumption. Carbohydrate-rich foods may also regulate the appetite, whereas foods rich in fat do not.

Alcohol

Because alcohol is toxic to the body, it will always be used as fast as the body can oxidize it and extract its calories. We burn the calories from alcohol first and then use up carbohydrates and proteins. Only then does the body get around to burning up fats.

This does *not* mean that the calories from beer or wine or bread don't count. These foods don't add to body fat directly, but if you don't want to gain weight or want to lose the fat you already have, reconsider taking a nip.

> **When you consume moderate amounts of alcohol or any carbohydrate food, it can stimulate your appetite, adding to the surplus of calories. Your body's need to**

**burn energy will be diverted from working off the fat
from either the last meal you had or the stores waiting
around the waist.**

Almost all chronic alcoholics who have a high caloric intake
from alcohol but eat little food are thin. In spite of this, many
of us cling to the idea that the typical beer gut is due to beer.
However, paunches of all sizes are composed of fat. Let's put
the blame where it deserves to be —on the food that is usually
consumed with beer.

Most beer drinkers eat fatty foods with their beer—peanuts,
deli meats, cheese, hamburgers, chips, fatty barbecues, and
large untrimmed steaks. It is rare to find anyone using the
amber liquid to wash down a green salad!

The reason many hearty drinkers get fat is that the fuel pro-
vided by alcohol is enough for their needs. Any calories from
fat consumed at the same time are therefore surplus and are
deposited as body fat—usually around the waist. A beer gut
should more correctly be called a *fat gut*.

Percentage of Calories from Fat

You may prefer to consider the percentage of calories that come
from fat rather than thinking in terms of grams of fat. For
example, many doctors are aiming to reduce our average fat
consumption from about 37 percent of energy to less than 30
percent. Some experts recommend an even stricter guideline of
no more than 10 percent of calories from fat.

If you had a detailed list of your food intake for the day, you
could calculate the number of grams of protein, fat, carbohydrate, and alcohol, and then work out what percentage of the
energy comes from each. This method is less appropriate to
work out an ideal energy percentage for any particular food and
would be a complicated daily undertaking that would require
more time and energy than the average person can spend.

One hundred percent of the energy in all foods must come from protein, fat, or carbohydrate. Foods that do not contain carbohydrates, such as meat or fish, must derive all of their calories from protein and fat. For example, a 4-ounce piece of fish has 2 grams of fat and 27 grams of protein. The 2 grams of fat provide 18 calories of energy and the protein provides 108. The total calories for that piece of fish is 135, of which fat provides 20 percent. If you wanted to follow a very low-fat diet, you might reject such fish, even though the absolute amount of fat is very low.

> **If you avoid adding a slurp of whole milk to your coffee or tea because of its high percentage of calories from fat, you are saving yourself only the negligible amount of half a gram.**

If you are concerned about controlling or losing body fat, it makes much more sense to aim for a particular number of grams of fat each day. If you want to lose weight, an intake of 30 to 40 grams is a good guideline to shoot for.

Fats Make Us Fat

Research now shows conclusively that fat in the diet is the major culprit in producing body fat. The body can store large amounts of fat. It is the last priority as a fuel for metabolism or physical activity. Eating more fat does not increase the amount of fat oxidized, and fat has little effect in satiating appetite. A diet high in fat leads to passive and chronic overconsumption, and increases the store of body fat.

> **There are many studies showing that body fat correlates with fat intake, not specifically with caloric intake.**

Of course, since fats have more than twice the caloric level of either carbohydrates or proteins, and a higher level than alcohol, a diet high in fat is usually high in calories. Americans eat a lot of fat. In spite of moves to low-fat dairy products and encouragement to trim fat from meat, fat consumption is still high, largely because of the high quantities of fat used in fast foods and processed foods.

Few people realize that they are eating a lot of fat. Many *think* they are eating less fat by consuming meals they consider "light." The composition of those foods show they are not light in fat. For example, a slice of quiche with salad can have six times the fat levels of lean meat and vegetables; a typical helping of lasagna can have far more fat than a traditional roast dinner.

> **Did you know that a fast food hamburger can contain up to 40 grams of fat compared with the 18 grams of the old-fashioned variety, or that spaghetti from your favorite restaurant has had every one of its strands of spaghetti coated in fat to prevent them sticking together and contains a rich cream-based sauce to boot!**

Meals eaten away from home almost always have more fat than those cooked in your kitchen. The influx of reduced-fat foods doesn't always help. There is some evidence that people maintain a liking for fat when they eat fat-reduced foods but lose their taste for it if they eat very little of it. Many reduced-fat products are still relatively high in fat. For example, reduced-fat margarines may have 60 percent fat, reduced-fat cheeses range from 7 to 25 percent fat (regular cheddar is 33 percent fat), and some reduced-fat pies and meals are still high in fat. Each of these products may have less fat than its regular counterpart but is still high in fat. Being labeled as "reduced-fat," however, may make people feel free to consume larger quantities. For example, you might hesitate to eat even one scoop of regular ice cream each night but may feel quite comfortable about frequently having two scoops of reduced-fat ice cream. It is much like putting skim milk in your coffee while scoffing apple pie with cream.

32

WINNING AT
WEIGHT LOSS

To lose fat, you'll need to know where dietary fats are hiding. You do not need to remove *all* fat from the diet—less will do nicely—and you can still allow foods to maintain flavor. Excess body fat accumulates because the calories entering the body from food and drink exceed the amount required for growth, physical activity, and metabolism. The only way to lose body fat is to create a calorie deficit until the excess fat is lost and then establish a balance between what comes in and what is used.

Genes and Your Jeans

Many people who are overweight are convinced they have some kind of deficiency in their metabolism. Many studies show this is rarely the case. The problem of excess body fat is almost always due to overconsumption and underactivity. Those who diet frequently, however, may be reducing lean tissue rather than fat, and lean tissue is what burns up calories twenty-four hours a day.

The role of genetics is continually being explored in nutritional research. One hundred years ago, obesity was rare.

> **Experts speculate that since our gene pool has changed very little since over the past century and technology has prevented many sweaty brows, most obesity is not primarily genetic.**

Some experts say that genes are responsible for only one-quarter to one-third of excess weight. Environmental factors such as food, drink, and exercise are still the major weight contributors. There is a common misconception that some people are fortunate enough never to gain weight. In fact, everyone will gain weight if overfed, but some will gain more than others. Either you or someone you know may seem to eat a lot but stay slim. This might be due to a tendency to eat more when others are present but not have a high intake overall. Some people are also natural fidgets who can burn up to 700 calories a day just in their constant body movements.

For those who need to lose body fat, here are some suggestions that might be useful, but note first these three important points:

- ❥ Not everyone is going to be the same size. No amount of dieting will give you sylphlike thighs if they don't run in your family. Remember that the health hazard is fat around the waist and on the upper body.
- ❥ Fast weight loss is not fat loss but represents mainly changes in the body's content of water, and some loss of lean tissue. Weight lost fast usually returns, often bringing a bonus 3 or 4 pounds.
- ❥ Changes in eating and exercise must be upheld forever, not just for three weeks or even three months or three years. Those changes therefore must be possible, sustainable, and enjoyable.

Sugars and Alcohol

The best way to create a calorie deficit is by eating less fat and doing more exercise to burn it up. Try also to reduce sugar and alcohol. Neither will directly add to body fat, but both are usually partnered with other fatty ingredients or other fatty foods. In addition, neither provides essential elements and both provide energy that the body could otherwise get from its fat stores. Trying to cut out sugar and alcohol, however, is not a good tactic, as forbidden foods become highly desirable. An occasional cake, chocolate, ice cream, or whatever sweet food you like makes good sense.

> **Make sure it is worth the calories by choosing an exceptional cake or chocolate rather than something mundane. You must also make sure that your "occasions" don't come more than once or twice a week.**

A daily glass of wine or a single beer won't usually interfere with successful fat loss, but don't consume it fast to satisfy thirst. No alcoholic beverage is a good thirst quencher, so always drink plenty of water *before* starting on any type of alcohol. Drinking one or two large glasses of water first is the most painless way to reduce alcohol consumption.

Fill 'er Up with Carbs

There is little point in cutting down on bulky carbohydrate foods. They have the great advantage of being filling. Most people can put up with feeling hungry for a day or so, but after that they become very hungry and less discriminating about what they eat. Many studies show that strict dieting leads to eating binges and greater consumption of high-fat foods. It makes more sense to eat foods such as potatoes, breads, cereals, and other grain products, as well as plenty of fruit and vegetables.

Eating fruit with fiber instead of drinking juice, and eating high-fiber bread, also helps to make you feel more satisfied. Most carbohydrate foods are served with something fatty, but there are many tasty alternatives. With just a smidgeon of imagination you can easily jazz up the flavor of your foods. Here are just a few ideas:

- Sprinkle on a teaspoon of olive oil and a bit of good Parmesan cheese. Both will impart far more flavor than bland oil or a large amount of mild cheese.

- Crisp up good-quality bread or rolls in a hot oven, or buy when very fresh so they taste good without a spread.

- Try pita and lavash breads with salad or hummus and tabouli, or with a variety of other ingredients.

- Dollop low-fat yogurt mixed with fresh snipped herbs on top of potatoes in place of butter.

- Serve or order steamed rice rather than fried rice.

- Make sauces for pasta by using a small amount of olive oil with low-fat ingredients such as tomatoes, mushrooms, eggplant, onions, garlic, herbs, wine, seafood, chicken breast, or very lean meat.

- Serve well-chilled fresh fruit in season, without cream or ice cream but with yogurt, if desired.

Weight-Loss Wisdom

Very strict diets don't work. Apart from the difficulty in sticking to them, eating very little carbohydrate leads to a loss of water and lean tissue and reduces the body's energy expenditure. Water losses can be replaced, but lean tissue burns up calories and its loss eventually leads to weight gain. If you try to follow a very low-calorie diet, your body reduces its energy expenditure—which is counterproductive. Eating very little and having low energy levels just make you feel awful. If you want to lose body fat, you will probably achieve success if you restrict your daily fat intake to 30 to 40 grams a day.

Fats and Oils

Fats and oils are major contributors to fat intake in this country.

Salad dressing is one of the primary source of dietary fat in women ages 19 to 50.

Fats and oils are used in the home for cooking and as spreads for bread. An even greater quantity come in processed and fast foods. Many of these foods are obviously fatty, leaving grease on your fingers. Others hide their fat in soft buns, meat patties coated with cheese, and fatty dressings added to make the product more moist so that it can be eaten more quickly.

Other high-fat foods include margarine, chips, doughnuts, cookies, chocolate and some other types of candy, cheeses, cakes, pastries, pies, croissants, and creamy sauces.

Attack the Snacks

Whether snacking is involved in weight gain is debatable. When given a set amount of food as either meals or snacks, most people burn more calories with the snacks. In practice, however, most people eat snacks in addition to their normal meals, and these become extra sources of fat and calories.

Americans spent $30 billion on snacks in 1999.

Perhaps the best example of the wisdom of avoiding snacks comes from France. Obesity is uncommon in France, even though the French people seem to eat many foods that the rest of the world regards as undesirable—for example, cheese and butter. Overall, the French do not snack a lot. Meals are taken so seriously that casual eating while walking along the street or driving in a car is less common than in countries such as ours, where meals and snacks mingle freely throughout the day. It is possible that the habit of eating discrete meals allows your body to digest one quantity of food and feel hungry before eating another. In other words, your body's natural appetite control mechanism works better than it does if you were to eat food merely in response to the sight of it.

Skip the Spreads

The average American reports eating 12 1/2 pounds of butter and margarine a year. If you were to skip the spreads, you could save yourself about 16 grams of fat a day. For big consumers, who are likely to be overweight, the saving will be even greater. In a recent study where people were asked to keep their total fat to 30 to 40 grams a day and were given a list of the fat content of foods but no other instructions, every person spontaneously decided that one of the easiest ways to reduce fat intake was to stop using margarine or butter. But changing to a reduced-fat spread does not usually work because most people simply use more. It takes only a week or so to become used to avoiding spreads. Eating bread with no spread is widely practiced in most Mediterranean countries, where bread consumption is two to four times greater than that of many other countries. It *is* possible, and almost certainly enjoyable.

Home Is Where the Health Is

It used to be that going outside of the home to eat or ordering takeout meals were viewed as special treats or celebrations. Today going out to eat is much more commonplace.

> In fact, the typical American spends about 46% of their food budget on meals outside of the home.

Almost without exception, fast foods are fatty and carry much higher fat levels than home-cooked foods do. For example, a typical fast food burger has 30 grams of fat; add another 20 grams if you eat it with a medium serving of French fries.

Fried chicken is no better, and 2 small slices of pizza can have 20 grams of fat. Add a salad with dressing and you've easily exceeded the day's 30-gram fat total in one small meal.

Adults and teenagers are now being wooed to eat fast food breakfasts too. This is another disaster, with a full breakfast of sausage, biscuit, and hash browns adding 40 grams of fat. Even scrambled eggs on an English muffin contribute 21 grams! Compare this with the total of 3 grams you get in a bowl of cereal with skim milk, some fresh fruit, and a slice of toast with jam.

The high-fat content of food eaten outside the home comes not only from the ingredients, but also from the larger-than-average serving sizes. This is more apparent at the lower price end of the market. Somewhat ironically, as you pay more, you get less. Our country is notorious in this respect.

> **A food or drink marked "small" is akin to something regarded as "giant-sized" in other countries. This undoubtedly contributes to our high levels of obesity.**

Fast food meals are seen as being quick, convenient, and relatively cheap, yet many meals can be prepared in 15 or 20 minutes at home from ingredients that can be stored in the pantry, fridge, and freezer and cost less than the total amount spent at a fast food restaurant. Some examples of quick and easy meals are listed in the next chapter.

Pull a Fast One on Fast Foods

Eat bread instead of crackers, cookies, pastries, or croissants.

Two average slices of bread or a fresh roll each have 1.5 grams of fat. A croissant can have as much fat as 19 slices of bread! A small pastry is similar. Crackers add up too. Six small crackers have 6 grams of fat, 1 cookie can have up to 13 grams of fat. As you would suspect, doughnuts are drenched in fat, with a small glazed doughnut weighing in at 14 grams. Imagine how lethal a doughnut becomes when you add cream filling and chocolate glaze.

Here are more ways to prune your diet:

Cut Fat off Meat and Chicken

Two lamb chops with fat have 30 grams of fat; trimmed of most external fat, they have 11 grams. Very lean meats now available have a low fat content and most cuts of chicken can now be found already skinned.

Choose Low-fat Milk and Yogurt

This is one of the easiest changes for most people. Low-fat milk won't save you much fat if you add only a few drops to your coffee or tea. However, if you drink it straight, use it on cereal or in cooking; it can really trim down your daily fat intake.

Use Plenty of Ingredients to Add Flavor to Foods

Herbs, spices, lemon, garlic, pepper, and wine have no fat, but adding them to food cooked without a lot of fat makes it taste much better. Extra-virgin olive oil can also add lots of flavor to a meal, but each teaspoon has 5 grams of fat, so always use it sparingly. All varieties of olive oil, including light, have the same fat and calorie level as any other oil.

In practice, you can keep fat to 30 to 40 grams, assuming servings are average size, as follows:

Food	Fat content (g)
Fruit, 3–6 pieces	<<1
Vegetables, 4–5 types	<<1
Bread, 6 slices	4
Breakfast cereal, 1 bowl	2

Skim milk or non-fat yogurt	0*
Regular milk in tea or coffee	4
Rice or pasta, 2 cups	2
Egg, cheese, or chicken breast sandwich	6
Lean meat or chicken, approx. 8 oz.	8**
Olive oil (in cooking), 1 Tsp.	5
Total	*33*

*If using 6 ounces of 2 percent reduced-fat milk, add 3.
**Substituting grilled seafood reduces this to 2 to 6 grams.

Frying in Fat

All fried foods absorb some fat. As discussed in Chapter 6, some oils should not be used more than once for frying because heat causes undesirable chemical changes in them. There are some misconceptions about frying, however, the greatest being that shallow-fried food absorbs less fat than deep-fried food.

The amount of fat absorbed depends on the type of food, the oil, and the frying temperature.

Some research has found that potato chips deep-fried at 356°F absorb 30 percent less fat than those cooked at lower temperatures.

Steak fries absorb less fat than thin French fries do. And Spanish and Italian researchers report that if you deep-fry in olive oil, less oil is absorbed into foods.

Most commercial deep-fried food is cooked in a highly saturated mixture of palm, palm kernel, and hydrogenated soybean or cottonseed oils. It may taste good, but it is a disaster for both your health and weight.

Polyunsaturated oils are not suitable for deep frying, as they are easily degraded by heat and can form undesirable compounds. The simplest solution is probably not to use them at all for deep frying.

33

Now You're Cooking!

Now you know that body fat serves some important functions and cell membranes, the brain, and other essential organs demand essential fatty acids that are found in the "good" fats you consume. Fats in your diet support the intricate workings of your body that help you motor along from one day to the next. Those same dietary fats can also accompany other important nutrients and protective factors in foods—for example, in nuts, avocado, seeds, soybeans, olive oil, fatty fish, and yogurt. Avoiding these foods because of their fat content could have adverse effects.

Fats in foods also carry flavor. This is vitally important because you are more likely to eat flavorful foods. If you try to cook without any fat, you won't enjoy the food for long. For example, you cannot get the same flavor from a steamed or boiled onion as you do when you fry the onion in some oil. Nor will low-fat ice cream have as much creamy taste as regular or premium ice cream.

However, the more-is-better school of thought doesn't apply to dietary fats. Some of the most innocent-looking meals can wreak havoc on your health. A restaurant can transform a simple cup of soup and a seemingly healthy bowl of salad into a disastrous dish swarming with saturated fats.

The good news is you don't need much fat to enhance the flavor of foods! An onion fried in two teaspoons of oil will have just as much flavor as one cooked in two tablespoons of oil. Succulent meals do not require vast quantities of fat. In fact, too much grease drowns the vibrant taste and texture of natural foods. Give your heart a break and try some of these quick and delicious meals that your taste buds (and your wallet) will appreciate.

Easy Eats (All Based on Average-Sized Servings)

Breakfasts (all with 3–4 grams of fat)

﹚ Cereal with fresh fruit, low-fat milk or yogurt, plus 1 slice of toast with honey or jam

﹚ Smoothie made with low-fat milk, 1–2 bananas, honey, and wheat germ

﹚ Pancake topped with yogurt and fresh blueberries

﹚ Oatmeal topped with raisins and brown sugar

Lunch (all less than 7 grams of fat)

﹚ Sliced turkey sandwich with cranberry sauce, plus 1–2 pieces of fruit

﹚ Lean chicken in pita bread with salad, plus 1 piece of fruit

﹚ Tuna or smoked salmon mixed with chopped celery and low-fat yogurt plus 1 roll, plus fruit

﹚ Homemade bean or vegetable soup with 1 dinner roll, plus fruit

﹚ Baked beans with 1 dinner roll

﹚ Large salad sprinkled with hard-boiled egg, 1 dinner roll, plus one or two pieces of fruit

Dinner (all less than 10–15 grams of fat, if cooked with very little oil)

﹚ Spaghetti with sauce made from tomatoes, garlic, mushrooms, eggplant, herbs, and red wine, plus a green salad dressed with balsamic vinegar and a few drops of olive oil

❱ Stir-fried pork with vegetables and rice

❱ Lean grilled beef with potato and vegetables

❱ Grilled fish, steamed or microwaved potatoes with parsley and chives, and salad or steamed or microwaved vegetables

❱ Couscous with grilled herbed chicken breast and vegetables stir-fried in a little olive oil

❱ Lasagna made with spinach and low-fat ricotta, plus a salad

Dessert

❱ fresh fruit of any kind, with low-fat yogurt if desired

Snacks (all less than 2 grams of fat)

❱ Fresh fruit of any kind

❱ Fresh bread (2 slices or one roll eaten plain)

❱ Milk shake made with low-fat milk, ice, low-fat yogurt, a little honey, and coffee, vanilla, or fresh fruit for flavor

❱ A container of low-fat yogurt

❱ Breakfast cereal with low-fat milk

❱ A couple of rice crackers with honey or banana

INDEX

ABOUT THE AUTHOR

ROSEMARY STANTON, Ph.D., is Australia's best-known nutritionist. She is the author of twenty-six books on food and nutrition, several thousand magazine and newspaper articles, and many scientific papers.